# PART ONE

# The Basics

# 1. What is cancer?

**Cells**

Microscopic units that make up the organs of the body.

Cancer is uncontrolled growth of **cells**—the billions upon billions upon billions of microscopic units that make up all the organs of our body. Cells are easily distinguished from each other. Lung cells are very different in appearance from colon cells, for example, and do very different things. Colon cells are very different from blood cells, which are very different from muscle cells, and so forth. To understand what cancer is, you must first understand what makes a normal cell normal.

Normal cells do their own thing. For example, red blood cells carry oxygen throughout the body, stomach cells absorb nutrients, and **white blood cells** fight infections.

**White blood cells**

A type of blood cell that fights infection.

Normal cells also stop growing and dividing when they get too old. In addition, normal cells often self-destruct (undergo **apoptosis**) and die if they are injured.

**Apoptosis**

Process by which normal cells die when they are injured; often referred to as programmed cell death.

Cancer cells differ from normal cells in a number of important ways. First, they are often unable to stop growing and dividing (unregulated growth). Second, cancer cells often stop doing their thing. In fact, they often stop doing anything useful at all. For example, cancerous white blood cells often stop fighting infection, stomach cancer cells stop absorbing nutrients, and lung cancer cells are unable to absorb oxygen. Another property of cancer cells is that they do not die like normal cells do when they grow old; they are literally immortal. In addition, cancer cells often spread to other organs, a process called **metastasis**. They can metastasize either by invading a nearby organ or by entering into the bloodstream or **lymphatic system** and traveling through the body to invade distant organs. Cancer cells can also make substances similar to hormones (called

**Metastasis**

The spread of cancer from the initial cancer site to other parts of the body.

**Lymphatic system**

A vascular system that contains lymph nodes through which white blood cells flow; cancer can also spread through the lymphatic system.

**growth factors**) which can stimulate other cancer or normal cells to grow.

A **tumor** is a mass of tissue formed by a new growth of cells. If a tumor stops growing by itself, and does not invade other tissues, it is considered **benign**. Examples include lipomas, which are soft, spongy, fatty tumors that form just under the skin. Most tumors are **malignant**, which means they exhibit all the properties of cancer cells we've just mentioned.

Cancer can vary widely in terms of the malignant features we've just described—both between different types of cancers (e.g., leukemia vs. prostate cancer vs. breast cancer), and between people with the same type of cancer. For example, some types of cancers are very fast growing (e.g., acute leukemia) whereas others are usually much more slow growing (e.g., chronic leukemia). Some types tend to spread early on in their course (e.g., small cell lung cancer) whereas others tend to invade adjacent tissues (e.g., soft tissue sarcomas). Some manage to retain some of the features of the tissues in which they arose (**well-differentiated** tumors) whereas others look so abnormal that the pathologist cannot tell where they came from by looking at them under a microscope (**poorly differentiated** tumors). Well-differentiated tumors tend to be slower growing and less aggressive, whereas poorly differentiated tumors often tend to grow and spread quickly. Thus, it is important that you realize that how someone else's breast cancer behaved, for example, is totally irrelevant to how your lung cancer is likely to behave—in terms of spread, growth rate, treatment, response to treatment, just about everything.

Just as different types of cancer vary in terms of how they behave (e.g., leukemia vs. prostate cancer vs. breast

---

**Growth factors**

Substances that stimulate cells to grow; drugs that help the bone marrow recover from the effects of chemotherapy.

**Tumor**

A mass of tissue formed by a new growth of cells.

**Benign**

Not cancerous; not life threatening.

**Malignant**

Cancerous; cells that exhibit rapid, uncontrolled growth and can spread to other parts of the body.

**Well-differentiated**

Cancer cells which look relatively similar to the organ in which they started.

**Poorly differentiated**

Cancer cells that look wildly abnormal and nothing like the organ they started in.

**THE BASICS**

cancer), the same type of cancer will vary in its behavior from person to person. For example, in some patients a lung cancer might tend to spread, or metastasize early on, whereas in others it might not spread for a long time. Also, even the same type of cancers varies in terms of how they respond to treatment. Chemotherapy can be highly effective in shrinking the tumor in some patients with lung cancer, for example, whereas in others, chemotherapy might just stop the cancer from growing or not work at all (the cancer could be totally resistant to it). Why cancers differ depending on the tumor type, and why cancers behave differently from patient to patient, is an area of great interest with lots of research going on.

## 2. How do normal lungs function?

Lungs are necessary for breathing—that is, bringing oxygen into the body and getting rid of carbon dioxide. Oxygen is necessary for cells to make energy. As this happens, the oxygen is used up and carbon dioxide is made. Carbon dioxide is a waste product, which needs to be removed from the body. This important oxygen–carbon dioxide exchange takes place in the lungs.

**Trachea**

Breathing tube (airway) leading from the larynx to the lungs.

**Main stem bronchi**

The two main breathing tubes (right main stem bronchus and left main stem bronchus) that branch off the trachea.

**Alveoli**

Tiny air sacs that compose the lungs.

When we breathe in, or inhale, air travels through the main breathing tube called the **trachea**, which divides into two tubes (**main stem bronchi**) in the area near the heart. One tube goes to the right lung (right main stem bronchus) and the other to the left (left main stem bronchus).

From there, the bronchi divide into smaller and smaller segments until they eventually become so tiny and thin that they are called alveoli. **Alveoli** are the millions of microscopic air sacs through which oxygen diffuses into red blood cells in the blood, where it is carried throughout the body. In exchange, carbon dioxide carried by the red blood cells from the body diffuses into the alveoli; it is then expelled out of the body through the airways when we exhale.

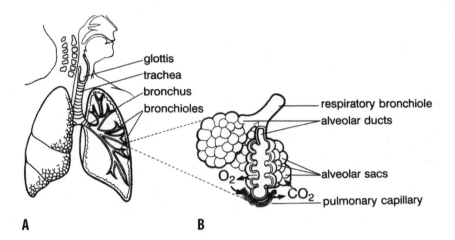

A

B

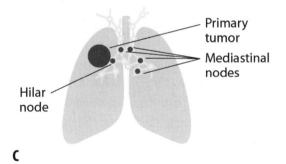

C

**Figure 1** Internal structure of the lungs.

**A.** Relationship of the lungs to the head and neck.

**B.** External and internal appearance of a lung lobule, showing the alveolar sacs.

**C.** Location of some representative hilar and mediastinal lymph nodes.

Parts A and B: Reprinted from Anderson PD and Spitzer VM. *Human Anatomy and Physiology Coloring Workbook and Study Guide, Third Edition.* Sudbury, MA: Jones and Bartlett Publishers, LLC, 2009.

Part C: Courtesy of the National Lung Cancer Partnership.

**Lobes**

Clear anatomical divisions or extensions that can be determined without the use of a microscope (at the gross anatomy level). The right lung contains three lobes and the left contains two.

**Lymph node**

Small collections of white blood cells scattered throughout the body.

**Hilar lymph nodes**

Lymph nodes located in the region where the bronchus meets the lung.

**Mediastinal lymph nodes**

Lymph nodes located in the mediastinum, the area between the lungs.

**N2 nodes**

Mediastinal nodes (e.g., nodes between the lungs and the heart).

**Squamous cell carcinoma**

A type of non-small cell lung cancer.

**Adenocarcinoma**

A type of non-small cell lung cancer; a malignant tumor that arises from glandular tissue.

Notice that each lung is divided into sections called **lobes**. The right lung has three lobes, but the left lung has only two to make room for the heart. The heart assists in the vital process of breathing by pumping blood to and from the lungs (**Figure 1**).

Also notice that there are **lymph nodes** in the lung and in the space between the heart and the lung. These are important because lung cancers tend to spread via the lymphatic system. It is important that the surgeon biopsy these lymph nodes because if they do have cancer in them it would change the prognosis and treatment (see Question 6). The most common lymph nodes are nodes in the lung (lobar nodes) or right where the lung begins (**hilar lymph nodes**), often called N1 nodes, or in the space between the lung and the heart (**mediastinal lymph nodes,** or **N2 nodes**).

## 3. Are there different types of lung cancer?

There are four major types of lung cancer: **squamous cell carcinoma**, **adenocarcinoma**, **large cell carcinoma**, and **small cell carcinoma**. The primary difference between squamous cell, adenocarcinoma, and large cell carcinoma is how they look under the microscope.

These three are sometimes collectively called **non-small cell lung cancer** (**NSCLC**) to distinguish them from **small cell lung cancer** (**SCLC**), or small cell carcinoma. In the United States, adenocarcinoma is the most common type of lung cancer, representing about 40% of all lung cancers. Sometimes, it is difficult to tell what type of NSCLC it is, in which case it might be called poorly differentiated or NSCLC—not otherwise specified (NSCLC-NOS).

Small cell lung cancer represents roughly 15%–20% of all lung cancers. It differs from the three types of non-small cell lung cancer in several important ways. It tends to be more rapidly growing, causes symptoms quicker, and spreads more rapidly. SCLC also tends to be more sensitive to **chemotherapy** and **radiation therapy** than NSCLC. For these reasons, patients with SCLC rarely undergo surgery. Instead, the standard treatment is chemotherapy, sometimes with radiation therapy (see Question 18).

Until very recently, squamous cell carcinoma, adeno-carcinoma, and large cell carcinoma were all treated the same way. However, more recent data suggest that some treatments might be more effective or safer in one sub-type than another.

One subtype of adenocarcinoma also bears mention-ing: **adenocarcinoma-in-situ** (**AIS**), formerly known as **bronchioloalveolar carcinoma** (**BAC**). AIS is a rare form of lung cancer, representing only about 5% of all lung cancers. For unknown reasons, the number of patients developing AIS is rising. AIS is unique in that it tends to spread diffusely throughout the alveoli (see Question 2), unlike the more typical lung cancer cells which tend to stick together and form solid, discrete masses. The cause of AIS is less clear than for other forms of lung cancer. AIS tends to occur in younger, nonsmoking women. Of all the types of lung cancer, it is the one that is most often found in patients who have never smoked, although it is also found in smokers.

**Large cell carcinoma**

A type of non-small cell lung cancer.

**Small cell carcinoma**

A type of lung can-cer that differs in appearance and behavior from non-small cell lung cancers (adenocarci-noma, squamous cell carcinoma, large cell carcinoma).

**Non-small cell lung cancer (NSCLC)**

A type of lung can-cer that includes adenocarcinoma, squamous cell carci-noma, and large cell carcinoma.

**Small cell lung cancer (SCLC)**

Refers to small cell carcinoma, as opposed to non-small cell lung cancers (adenocarci-noma, squamous cell carcinoma, large cell carcinoma).

**Chemotherapy**

The use of medicine to treat cancer; a whole-body or sys-temic treatment.

**Radiation therapy**

Treatment that uses high-dose X-rays or other high-energy rays to kill cancer cells.

THE BASICS

**Adenocarcinoma-in-situ (AIS)**

Formerly called bronchioloalveolar carcinoma, a subtype of adenocarcinoma sometimes found in non-smokers.

**Bronchiolo-alveolar carcinoma (BAC)**

Now called adeno-carcinoma-in-situ (AIS); a type of adenocarcinoma.

**Passive smoking**

Inhaling cigarette smoke of others.

# 4. What causes lung cancer? Who gets lung cancer?

Eighty-five to 90% of lung cancers are caused by carcinogens in tobacco that cause damage (mutations) to the DNA in lung cells. People are usually exposed to these carcinogens by directly inhaling them while smoking; however, people can sometimes develop lung cancer because they have inhaled large quantities of smoke from other smokers (**passive smoking**). Rarely, radon (a gas found underground) can also cause lung cancer. Exposure to asbestos, air pollution, and certain other environmental carcinogens can also cause lung cancer. When this occurs, it is usually a result of long-term, occupational exposure. However, sometimes people who have never smoked and do not have a history of exposure to any of these environmental carcinogens also get lung cancer. More research is needed to determine why these individuals get lung cancer. It is not inherited, in the sense that your parents cannot pass down an abnormal gene to you that will make you get lung cancer, and you cannot pass an abnormal gene to your children that will give them lung cancer. (Unlike some other cancers, such as breast cancer, which in some cases can be inherited.) Even mutated genes we know cause lung cancer, such as EGFR or ALK, cannot be passed down from generation to generation. However, scientists are trying to determine if smokers can inherit an increased susceptibility to developing lung cancer. This might explain why some people who smoke develop lung cancer, while others do not.

**Incidence**

The number of new cases of a cancer (or any disease or event) in a defined population during a set period of time.

Lung cancer is second only to prostate cancer in men and breast cancer in women in **incidence** (the number of new patients who develop a cancer in 1 year per 100,000 people). Unfortunately, lung cancer is the leading cause of cancer death among both men and women and is responsible for more cancer-related deaths than breast cancer, colon cancer, and prostate cancer combined.

Lung cancer is most commonly found in current or former smokers, usually in their late 60s. The incidence of lung cancer has been on the rise since smoking became popular in the 1920s and 1930s, but it began to rise rapidly around 1960 when the effects of the cigarette boom during the World War II years became evident. The death rate for lung cancer in men peaked in the late 1980s; however, it continued to rise in women until roughly the year 2000, when it started to level off. Many people do not realize that lung cancer is the leading cancer killer of both men and women. Of note, although stopping smoking significantly decreases the risk of lung cancer, the risk never goes down to zero. Approximately 50% of all lung cancers occur in former smokers. This does not mean that it does not matter if one quits smoking or not. Even if the risk of lung cancer never goes down to zero, it still drops precipitously. In addition, there are multiple other health benefits to quitting smoking, such as a reduction in heart disease, high blood pressure, and other health problems.

For reasons we do not understand, occasionally people who have never smoked get lung cancer. An estimated 15% of lung cancer patients in the United States have never smoked. In certain areas of the world, the percentage is much higher. For example, in Asia the majority of women who get lung cancer have never smoked.

# PART TWO

# Diagnosis and Staging

## 5. What are the most common symptoms of lung cancer?

The symptoms of lung cancer depend upon its location. If a cancer occurs near the center of the chest, for example, it often presses on a major airway or blood vessel. In these cases, common symptoms include cough (including blood-tinged **sputum**) and shortness of breath. If the tumor blocks or obstructs a major airway, bacteria and secretions can back up behind the obstruction, resulting in a post-obstructive **pneumonia**.

Other structures near the center of the chest are sometimes affected by lung cancer. Rarely, the recurrent laryngeal nerve might be involved. The recurrent laryngeal nerve is a nerve that goes from the brain to the vocal cords. Because of the way humans develop as fetuses, this nerve does not make a direct path from the brain to the vocal cord as one might expect. Instead, it travels down to the chest and then back up again, swinging by the major vessels leading in and out of the heart. If the tumor happens to press upon this nerve, hoarseness can result. Similarly, if the tumor happens to press on the **esophagus**, the feeding tube that leads from the mouth to the stomach, patients can experience problems with swallowing. If the tumor presses on one of the great vessels leading into the heart, such as the superior vena cava, the blood sometimes cannot flow easily into the heart. Instead, it backs up into the neck, shoulders, and arms (**superior vena cava syndrome [SVCS]**). In this case, patients can experience swelling of these areas.

If the tumor arises farther out in the lung near the chest wall, patients can experience pain. Indeed, this is often the only time patients experience pain from lung cancer, because this is really the only area of the lung that has

**Sputum**

Mucus and other secretions produced by the lungs.

**Pneumonia**

An infection of the lung.

**Esophagus**

The tube through which food travels from the mouth to the stomach.

**Superior vena cava syndrome (SVCS)**

A collection of symptoms that could include swelling in the neck, shoulders, and arms caused by a lung tumor pressing on the SVC, one of the large vessels leading into the heart.

nerve endings. The middle of the lung and the area near the heart do not have many nerve endings, so tumors that arise in these areas rarely cause pain. This is one of the reasons why lung cancer can grow unnoticed for a long period of time, since it is often painless unless the chest wall is involved. Tumors arising near the chest wall can also cause a **pleural effusion** (see Question 23). A pleural effusion is an accumulation of fluid between the outside of the lung and the inside of the chest wall. This fluid can cause pain, cough, and shortness of breath.

If the tumor occurs near the top of the lung (**Pancoast tumor** or **superior sulcus tumor**), it could grow into some of the nerves leaving the spinal cord and travel down through the armpit and into the arm. In this case, it can cause shoulder pain or weakness, or an unusual group of symptoms consisting of a droopy eyelid, dry eyes, and lack of sweating on the face.

If the tumor metastasizes, its symptoms will be related to the area of the body to which it has spread. For example, if the cancer spreads to the bone, it could cause pain in the back, hip, leg, or arm. If it spreads to the brain, it can cause headaches, nausea, or signs and symptoms similar to a stroke. These symptoms are not unique to metastatic lung cancer—any cancer that spreads to these organs will cause similar symptoms. The most frequent symptoms of cancer, however, are fatigue, weakness, loss of appetite, and weight loss. These symptoms often indicate that the cancer is advanced.

**Pleural effusion**

Accumulation of fluid between the outside of the lung and the inside of the chest wall.

**Pancoast tumor (superior sulcus tumor)**

A tumor occurring near the top of the lungs that may cause shoulder pain or weakness or a group of symptoms including a droopy eyelid, dry eyes, and lack of sweating on the face.

**Superior sulcus tumor**

See Pancoast tumor.

## 6. How is lung cancer diagnosed? Which tests are performed to diagnose lung cancer?

The diagnosis of lung cancer frequently is made when a patient goes to his or her primary care physician complaining of cough, shortness of breath, and low-grade fevers. Because these symptoms are so common, the patient is often treated for bronchitis or respiratory infection with antibiotics without taking a chest **X-ray**. If the symptoms do not go away, however, a chest X-ray is eventually obtained, revealing some type of mass in the chest. The X-ray is frequently followed by a chest CT scan to provide a better picture of the lungs and chest. This, in turn, often results in a **biopsy** (sampling of tissue), which is required for diagnosis of any type of cancer.

A computed tomography, or CT scan (sometimes called a CAT scan), is the most helpful test for visualizing an abnormality in the lung. CT scans are a series of X-rays in which the body is sliced up like a loaf of bread. Each one of the slices is then called up on a computer screen to give a cross-sectional image of the chest. A CT scan offers considerably more detail than a regular chest X-ray. To help the radiologist distinguish between blood vessels and tumors on CT scans, a dye called CT or IV contrast is sometimes injected into the vein to make the blood vessels more pronounced.

Once a suspicious abnormality is found on a CT scan, the patient needs a biopsy to obtain a diagnosis. There are several ways of doing this:

- **Bronchoscopy**. A bronchoscopy is a procedure in which a lung doctor (**pulmonologist**) inserts a

**X-ray**
High-energy radiation used to image the body.

**Biopsy**
Removal of tissue or fluid sample for microscopic examination.

**Bronchoscopy**
A procedure that involves inserting a flexible tube (bronchoscope) through the nose down into the lungs. Needles can be inserted through the bronchoscope to obtain biopsy samples.

**Pulmonologist**
A physician who specializes in the diagnosis and treatment of lung diseases.

flexible tube called a **bronchoscope** through the nose down into the lungs. The bronchoscope, which has fiber optic lighting inside, has several purposes. It can serve as a periscope, allowing the pulmonologist to see into the airways. Additionally, needles can be inserted through the bronchoscope to obtain biopsies. The procedure is usually done on an outpatient basis, under sedation.

Although bronchoscopy is a commonly used diagnostic test, it does have several disadvantages. First, the pulmonologist usually cannot get the tube into the distant areas of the lung—the airways near the chest wall are too small for the bronchoscope to get through. Therefore, the use of this test is limited to the larger bronchi, or airways. Second, if the cancer itself is not actually growing in the airway, it can be difficult for the pulmonologist to get a biopsy because he or she cannot actually see the tumor.

## Alternatives

- **Transthoracic (percutaneous) biopsy.** Specialized doctors, called **interventional radiologists**, can sometimes insert a needle from the outside in—through the skin and chest wall into the tumor—in order to obtain tissue for a biopsy. This procedure usually does not require a hospital stay (it is an outpatient procedure) and is often done under a local anesthetic.

- **Surgery.** Sometimes the abnormality seen on chest X-ray or CT scan cannot be easily biopsied by either a bronchoscopy or a transthoracic biopsy. In this case, patients might have to undergo a relatively minor surgical procedure under a general anesthetic (and thus might require an overnight stay in the hospital).

**DIAGNOSIS AND STAGING**

**Bronchoscope**
See bronchoscopy.

**Transthoracic (percutaneous) biopsy**

A biopsy in which a needle is inserted from the outside into the tumor.

**Interventional radiologist**

A radiologist who uses X-rays and other imaging techniques to perform minimally invasive medical procedures.

**Surgery**

Removal of tissue by means of an operation (surgical procedure).

*15*

The surgeon can do several different procedures to make the diagnosis. These include:

**Mediastinoscopy**

A surgical procedure by which lymph nodes can be removed for microscopic examination.

**Mediastinum**

Area between the lungs.

**Video-assisted thoracoscopic surgery (VATS)**

A type of minimally invasive chest surgery.

**Robotic surgery**

A type of minimally invasive surgery, in which the surgeon manipulates the instruments from a console that does not have to be next to the patient's bed.

– **Mediastinoscopy**. This procedure involves making a small incision above the collarbone or between the spaces of the first and second or second and third ribs. The surgeon then inserts a special tube through this incision into the **mediastinum**. Again, this tube has two functions: it allows the surgeon to see the lymph nodes near the heart, and it also allows the surgeon to biopsy them. A mediastinoscopy is sometimes done not only to make the diagnosis of cancer but also to help stage the patient (see Question 7).

– **Video-assisted thoracoscopic surgery (VATS)**. This procedure involves making a small incision someplace on the outside of the chest and inserting a fiber optic tube into the space between the chest wall and the lung. This allows a surgeon to see the outside of the lung and to biopsy any suspicious areas.

– **Robotic surgery**. No, this does not mean the surgery is carried out by a robot! This is similar to a VATS procedure except the fiber optic instruments are smaller. The surgeon manipulates the instruments from a console that doesn't have to be next to the patient's bed.

## 7. What is staging? What are the staging guidelines for NSCLC and SCLC?

**Staging**

Determining the size of a cancer and how far it has spread.

**Staging** a tumor involves determining where the tumor is, its size, and how far a cancer has spread. This is useful for several reasons:

- Staging allows physicians to have a common language in describing a patient's tumor. Thus, when a surgeon tells an oncologist that a patient has Stage IIIA lung cancer, the oncologist immediately has some idea as to the extent of the patient's disease.

- It is an important prognostic indicator. Patients with Stage I disease, for example, typically do much better than do patients with Stage IV disease.

- It is very useful for determining therapy. The type of treatment that is recommended—surgery, radiotherapy, chemotherapy, or any combination of these—will depend upon the extent of the disease and how far it has spread.

## Staging Guidelines for Non-Small Cell Lung Cancer (NSCLC)

The staging of cancer is classically dependent upon three criteria: the size and location of the tumor (T or tumor status), whether any lymph nodes are involved (N or nodal status), and whether the cancer has spread further than the lymph nodes (M or metastatic status). These three criteria (T, N, and M) are further subdivided. For example, if no lymph nodes contain the tumor, this is called N0; if the local (hilar) lymph nodes contain the tumor, this is called N1; and if the lymph nodes between the lung and the heart (mediastinal lymph nodes) contain tumor, this is typically called N2. N3 disease involves the lymph nodes in the other side of the chest or in the area above the collar bone.

Oncologists use a complicated system, based upon the TNM staging, to determine the overall stage. A simplified summary is provided in **Table 1**.

**Table 1** Lung Cancer Staging Based upon the TNM Staging Criteria

| | |
|---|---|
| **Stage 0** | Cancer is limited to the lining of the air passages and has not yet invaded the lung tissue. |
| **Stage I** | Cancer has invaded the underlying lung tissue, but has not yet spread to the lymph nodes. |
| **Stage II** | Cancer has spread to the neighboring lymph nodes or has spread to the chest wall, or the diaphragm, or the pleura between the lungs, or membranes surrounding the heart. |
| **Stage III** | Cancer has spread from the lung to either the lymph nodes in the center of the chest or the collarbone area. The cancer may have spread locally to areas such as the heart, blood vessels, trachea, and esophagus. |
| **Stage IV** | Cancer has spread to other parts of the body, such as the liver, bones, or brain. Cancer cells are found in the fluid around the lungs and heart (malignant pleural effusion and malignant pericardial effusion). |

## Staging Guidelines for Small Cell Lung Cancer (SCLC)

Because SCLC tends to metastasize early, oncologists typically do not go into the formal TNM staging classification noted above. Instead, they typically divide SCLC into limited stage or extensive stage disease, in which limited stage is defined as cancer confined to one side of the chest, and extensive stage is defined as cancer that has spread outside the side of the chest from which it arose.

The most common metastatic sites for both non-small cell and small cell lung cancer are in the lungs, the liver, the adrenal glands, the bones, and the brain.

# 8. Who treats lung cancer? What is multidisciplinary care?

Lung cancer is a complex disease, and its treatment frequently involves some combination of surgery, chemotherapy, and radiation (see Questions 12, 13, and 18). You likely will see more than one specialist for your lung cancer care, including medical oncologists, thoracic surgeons, radiation oncologists, and pulmonologists. Ideally, these lung cancer doctors work together in a **multidisciplinary clinic** or other setting where they can easily consult together, with each other, about your treatment options. This multidisciplinary approach not only offers you high-quality care but also has practical advantages that might include fewer trips to the doctor, less time from diagnosis to start of treatment, and more efficient coordination of the logistics involving treatment. Multidisciplinary care is commonly offered in cancer centers and in larger treatment centers such as university hospitals, but it is beginning to be implemented in some community hospitals as well.

Each lung cancer specialist you see is a member of your treatment team, but one doctor (usually the medical oncologist) will have primary responsibility for managing and directing your care.

There are also a number of other doctors, along with support staff, who will be involved in your care. It is helpful to understand what each of these healthcare professionals does and what role he or she plays in your care.

- *Medical oncologist*: a physician who performs comprehensive management of cancer patients throughout all phases of care. Medical oncologists specialize in treating cancer with medicine, using **systemic** treatments such as chemotherapy.

**Multidisciplinary clinic**

A multidisciplinary clinic is one in which doctors of different specialities (e.g., medical oncology, radiation oncology, and surgeons) all see the patient within the same clinic.

**Systemic**

Affecting the entire body.

- *Thoracic surgeon*: a surgeon who specializes in performing lung surgery. A thoracic surgeon might have performed the tumor biopsy that resulted in your lung cancer diagnosis. Some thoracic surgeons have received additional training in lung cancer surgery and are considered surgical oncologists.

- *Radiation oncologist*: a physician who specializes in treating cancer with radiation.

- *Pulmonologist*: a physician who specializes in the diagnosis and treatment of lung diseases. A pulmonologist might have diagnosed your lung cancer. You could also see a pulmonologist if you have ongoing respiratory issues related to your lung cancer or underlying conditions such as bronchitis, emphysema, or **chronic obstructive pulmonary disease (COPD)**.

**Chronic obstructive pulmonary disease (COPD)**

Emphysema and chronic bronchitis are the two most common forms of COPD.

Other specialists or support staff include:

- *Pathologist*: a physician trained to examine and evaluate cells and tissue under the microscope. The pathologist evaluates your biopsy tissue and furnishes a biopsy report to your oncologist or surgeon.

- *Oncology nurse*: a specialized nurse trained to provide care to cancer patients, including administering chemotherapy and monitoring side effects.

- *Psychiatrist*: a physician who specializes in treating people for depression, anxiety, and other psychological illness. Psychiatrists provide psychotherapy and can also prescribe medication.

- *Psychologist*: a person trained in psychology who can provide psychotherapy or counseling to help patients and their families better cope with their disease.

- *Patient navigator*: a nurse, nurse practitioner, social worker, or other healthcare personnel whose job is to coordinate your care (make sure all your questions are answered, your tests are scheduled, your treatments are on time, etc.) If your hospital or doctor's office is lucky enough to have a patient navigator, get this person's phone number! He or she will probably be your primary point person.

- *Oncology social worker*: a social worker trained to provide counseling and practical assistance to cancer patients. Social workers can help you locate services such as transportation, support groups, and home care. They can also provide assistance with insurance and financial issues.

- *Rehabilitation specialist*: a person trained to help patients recover from physical changes brought about by cancer or cancer treatment. Respiratory therapists help lung cancer patients to maximize their breathing capacity and learn to cope with breathlessness. Physical therapists can help patients recover range of motion and strength following lung cancer surgery.

- *Nutritionist* or *dietician*: a person trained to provide nutritional or dietary counseling. Lung cancer patients could experience weight loss as a result of their cancer or its treatment (see Question 24). Treatment side effects, such as nausea from chemotherapy or heartburn from radiation, can negatively affect appetite. Nutritional or dietary counseling services can help patients to increase appetite and gain weight.

- *Palliative care specialist*: a physician trained in managing cancer pain and other symptoms of cancer.

## 9. How can I relate best to my doctor? What can I do to make my medical visits as productive as possible?

The doctor–patient relationship lies at the heart of patient care. This relationship will guide and support you throughout the course of your lung cancer. It is your job, and your doctor's, to nurture this relationship and to work toward a partnership based on mutual trust and respect. Although difficulties between doctor and patient can occur at times, just as they do in any relationship, these problems will be minimized if good communication is maintained. Remember that your doctor is not a mind reader. It is your responsibility to be open and honest and to bring up any concerns, needs, or preferences you might have. It is especially important that you feel comfortable discussing sensitive issues, such as your use of alternative medicine treatments, your lifestyle (smoking, drinking, drugs), end-of-life issues, and sexual concerns. Keep in mind that conversations between doctor and patient are confidential (your family does not need to know if you don't want them to) and that the more your doctor knows about issues that could impact your health, the better care you will receive.

At your first visit you should address the issues of how much information you want from your doctor and how involved you would like to be in the decisions that are made about your care. Some patients want to know everything about their condition, and they want to make all the decisions themselves. Some patients find too much information anxiety-provoking. These patients would prefer to hear less information (or only the good news) and are more comfortable allowing their doctor to make all the decisions. Most patients fall somewhere in between. Whatever your preferences might be, and they can change over time, you need to communicate them to your doctor. If you feel that your doctor is not responsive to your needs, or if you have other concerns regarding your relationship, you should bring them up before they reach a crisis stage. If you and your doctor cannot resolve disagreements in a productive and satisfactory manner, you should look for another doctor.

It is also important to discuss with your doctor how much you do or do not want your family involved. If you do not want your doctor discussing your case with family members without you present, tell your doctor. Most doctors will ask you to sign a release of information form, giving them permission to talk to whomever you designate, before they will talk to a friend or family member when you are not around.

Think about what you are going to say to your doctor ahead of time. Remember, he or she has a certain amount of time to spend with you. Before your appointment consider which concerns are most pressing and write them down in order of importance. This tactic will help you focus and make the most effective use of the limited time you have with your doctor. Too often, patients spend their time with the doctor trying to remember if the pain started "on Monday when Aunt Ellie was visiting for dinner, or on Tuesday afternoon when they went out shopping, or Tuesday morning before breakfast, or maybe Wednesday when Aunt Ellie came back to pick up the casserole dish she forgot." If you choose to review events in great detail, you risk running out of the time that your doctor has for addressing more important issues.

If you have symptoms to report, describe them clearly and concisely. Be prepared to answer your doctor's questions, such as when the symptoms started, how often they occur, and how long they last. In most instances, you do not have to be exact; saying "early last week" or "about 2 months ago" will suffice. Don't be afraid to mention the emotional and social issues that are affecting you, in addition to any physical problems you have.

Always bring someone with you to your appointment. It is impossible to remember all that is said during an office visit, and emotions can cloud what a patient hears. It helps to have someone else along who can write down what the doctor says. Audio or video recording your conversations is another very helpful way of remembering exactly what transpired. As long as you tell the doctor what you are doing, most physicians have no problem with this. It is important that you understand everything that your doctor tells you. If something is unclear, say so, and ask questions until you are satisfied that you understand completely.

Many oncologists have an oncology nurse, nurse practitioner, or patient navigator with whom they work closely. *Get this person's name and number!* He or she can answer a lot of questions the doctor might not have time for, particularly between visits, and is often your patient advocate with your doctor. In many cases, he or she will be the go-between for you and your doctor, particularly between visits when problems or questions come up.

Be sure that all necessary tests are completed prior to your visit and that you have all the information you need. This includes having the required referrals, if any, and a current list of the prescription and nonprescription drugs you are taking. (It is very helpful to *bring the actual pill bottles along with you during EACH visit.*) Bring a notebook or binder that contains your medical information and paperwork to each appointment. If you can present your doctor with the information he or she needs to care for you in an efficient and clear manner, you will go a long way toward increasing the quality of your relationship with your doctor and, ultimately, the quality of your care.

## 10. How do I regain control of my life after my lung cancer diagnosis? How do I get past the emotional impact and move forward?

A lung cancer diagnosis can be overwhelming, making it difficult to absorb information and focus on what needs to be done. Your mind might be clouded with thoughts and worries about what your lung cancer will mean for you and your family. To move forward effectively, you need to make a mental adjustment. You need to redirect your energies toward the things you can control. Although you cannot change the fact that you have lung cancer, you can control how you respond to this challenge.

A first step toward gaining control of your thoughts is to realize that you are not alone in facing lung cancer. Thousands of people are surviving with lung cancer and leading happy, productive lives. The National Coalition for Cancer Survivorship defines a cancer survivor as anyone with a diagnosis of cancer, and you are considered a survivor from the moment of diagnosis. Cancer is not a death sentence. Many people view cancer as a chronic disease, something to be treated and managed. Keeping this concept in mind will help make your cancer experience less frightening.

Try to focus your energies on the following activities:

- *Adopting a healthy lifestyle.* Not smoking, maintaining adequate nutrition, and minimizing stress can all help your ability to fight your disease and withstand the effects of your cancer treatment.

- *Assembling a medical team.* You need to find doctors whom you can trust and who will provide you with excellent care. This could involve getting second opinions. You should keep in mind that good communication with all members of your medical team—including support personnel—is critical to the quality of care you receive (see Question 8).

- *Gathering information and making informed decisions.* You need to learn all you can about lung cancer and its treatment so that you will understand what is happening to you. After gathering information and discussing your treatment options with your doctor, you will be able to make informed decisions about your care.

- *Learning to navigate the healthcare system.* Your doctor's office staff and hospital social workers can help you learn how to navigate the healthcare system. This will make your appointments more productive and minimize the aggravation over medical paperwork, insurance, and financial concerns.

Consider joining a patient advocacy group. There are several specific to lung cancer and you can research the various groups to find one whose mission best fits your interest. For example, you might try research, fundraising, patient support, education/awareness, or legislative initiatives (see Appendix).

# PART THREE

# *Treatment Options*

## 11. What types of treatments are available for lung cancer?

The three traditional treatments for lung cancer include surgery, radiation therapy, and chemotherapy. Lung surgery commonly involves an operation to remove the tumor, along with nearby lymph nodes (see Question 12). Radiation therapy, or **radiotherapy**, is the delivery of a beam of radiation aimed at the tumor with the goal of killing some or all of the cancer cells, thus shrinking the tumor (see Question 18). Both surgery and radiotherapy are local forms of treatment, which means that they kill or remove only the tumor they are aimed at. Chemotherapy is a word for medications that kill cancer cells or stop their growth (see Question 13). Most chemotherapies are given **intravenously** (injected or dripped into the veins), but some are pills and are given orally. In either case, they get into the bloodstream and circulate around the body. Because blood flows through all parts of the body, in theory, cancer cells anywhere in the body would be exposed to the chemotherapy. Therefore, chemotherapy is a systemic therapy. Recently, **targeted therapy** has been added as a fourth modality for lung cancer. Targeted therapies are oral or intravenous medications that target abnormalities found specifically in tumors or cancer cells but not most normal tissues. Although targeted therapies are systemic treatments, like chemotherapy, they tend to have different side effects.

New treatments for lung cancer are always being tested in research studies known as clinical trials. You should familiarize yourself with the advantages and disadvantages of participation in clinical trials and explore the treatment options available to you through clinical trials (see Question 20). If you are considering alternative

**Radiotherapy**

The treatment of disease with ionizing radiation. Also called radiation therapy.

**Intravenous**

In the vein.

**Targeted therapy**

Therapy directed at aspects of the cell that are specific for cancer.

therapies, such as herbal therapies, you should have an understanding of how to evaluate them. Alternative therapies are treatments not endorsed by the traditional medical establishment because their effectiveness and safety have not been proven in rigorous scientific studies.

# 12. What is surgery for lung cancer? What determines whether I am able to have surgery and how is it performed? What should I expect following surgery?

Ideally, surgery for lung cancer should be done by a thoracic surgeon (see Question 8). The type of surgery performed depends upon the stage of tumor, and the medical condition of the patient.

To determine whether a patient is a candidate for surgery, three things must be established first:

1. Has the cancer metastasized? If the cancer has spread to other organs (Stage IV), a surgical cure is not possible and it does not make sense to do a large operation, considering the side effects, cost, and risks associated with surgery. Therefore, patients with metastatic disease usually do not undergo a curative resection.

2. The tumor must be **resectable**—that is, located in a place that the surgeon will be able to get to and completely remove. For example, if the tumor involves the heart, the surgeon obviously cannot safely remove the heart, and the tumor would be considered unresectable. In general, a tumor is considered unresectable if it involves any other major structures in the center of the chest, such

**Resectable**

Able to be surgically removed (resected).

as the heart, the large blood vessels going in and out of the heart, or the windpipe leading from the mouth to the lungs (the trachea).

3. The third criterion for surgery is that a patient must be healthy enough to withstand it. In particular, this involves two organs—the heart and the lungs.

    a. If you have a history of heart disease, such as congestive heart failure, angina, or heart attacks, your surgeon will want to make sure that it is safe to operate on you, so that the stress of the surgery will not result in a heart attack. He or she might ask you to see a cardiologist, or heart doctor. The cardiologist will take a history, examine you, and might order an electrocardiogram (EKG), echocardiogram, or stress test before giving a final recommendation.

    b. Many patients with lung cancer are smokers or former smokers and have some degree of emphysema or bronchitis (also known as chronic obstructive pulmonary disease, or COPD). If your doctor suspects you have COPD, he or she will order **pulmonary function tests** (**PFTs**). PFTs are a series of breathing tests that can help determine how healthy your lungs are and whether your remaining lungs will be able to support you if a portion of one of them has been removed. Your doctor might also order a preoperative quantitative perfusion scan, which is a nuclear medicine scan designed to predict how much lung function you will be left with after the operation.

**Pulmonary function tests (PFTs)**

A group of breathing tests used to determine lung health.

The most typical operation is a lobectomy and mediastinal **lymph node dissection**. A **lobectomy** is the removal of the lobe of the lung in which the tumor is located. A mediastinal lymph node dissection consists of removing some or all of the mediastinal lymph nodes (the lymph nodes between the lung and heart). This is often done to determine whether the tumor has spread to these lymph nodes. Occasionally, a patient might be unable to tolerate a lobectomy because underlying bronchitis or emphysema (COPD) makes it too difficult for the remaining lung to keep the person alive. In these cases, a surgeon will sometimes do a **wedge resection**. This consists of removing the tumor and a small amount of lung tissue surrounding the tumor, but not the whole lobe. A wedge resection will preserve more normal lung, but the chances of the cancer coming back are somewhat higher.

Occasionally, the tumor is located in an area such that all the lobes of the lung on that side are involved, meaning that they all contain some tumor. Sometimes the tumor is located in the largest airway on that side (the right or left main stem bronchus, which is the first major division of the trachea, the air pipe that delivers air to the lungs). If one of the main stem bronchi is involved, or if the tumor involves all the lobes on one side, a **pneumonectomy** must be performed. In a pneumonectomy, the whole lung is removed. Obviously, this is a much bigger procedure than a lobectomy or a wedge resection. Although a person with two normal lungs should be able to tolerate removal of one of the lungs without a major impact on his or her breathing, very often patients who have been smoking and have a substantial amount of emphysema or bronchitis are not able to tolerate a pneumonectomy.

**Lymph node dissection**
Surgical removal of lymph nodes.

**Lobectomy**
Surgical removal of a lobe of the lung.

**Wedge resection**
Surgical removal of the tumor and a small amount of lung tissue surrounding the tumor.

**Pneumonectomy**
Surgical removal of the entire lung.

TREATMENT OPTIONS

**Thoracotomy**

A common type of lung surgery that requires a large incision to provide access to the lungs.

**Minimally invasive surgery**

Surgery which uses smaller incisions than a regular operation and thus is less painful for the patient post-operatively. In order to be able to operate through such a small incision, the surgeon must use advanced, fibro electronic instruments.

**Patient-controlled analgesia (PCA)**

A method by which a patient can regulate the amount of pain medication he or she receives.

Typically, lung surgery involves an operation called a **thoracotomy**, which requires the surgeon to make a large incision in the chest to gain access to the lungs. Video-assisted thoracoscopic surgery (VATS) is an example of a less invasive surgical technique (also called **minimally invasive surgery**), which involves smaller incisions and therefore reduced post-operative pain and complications and shorter hospital stays. Robotic surgery is another form of minimally invasive surgery, in which the surgeon manipulates the instruments via a computer screen.

## Following Surgery

When you wake up in the recovery room, you will be very woozy and might not realize where you are, or even that the operation is over. You will doze off and on while you are brought back to your room. If possible, it is often helpful to have a family member or loved one stay with you during those first few days. He or she can call the nurses for you, help make you comfortable, and assist you in getting around.

For the first 24 to 48 hours, you could be uncomfortable, but the nurses should respond to your request for pain medications. Ask your doctor if you can have **patient-controlled analgesia** (**PCA**), a method by which you can regulate your own pain medication. By pressing a button attached to an IV, you can give yourself a small dose of morphine whenever you need it so that you do not have to wait for a nurse. The PCA machine is set so that you will not be able to overdose yourself.

You most likely will have a chest tube when you come out of surgery. This is a tube leading from the space between your lung and chest wall to a bag or container by your bedside. Suction is applied to drain the fluid and inflate the lung. Fortunately, this is not as painful or uncomfortable as it sounds! In addition, you will probably have a catheter leading from your bladder to a bag by the bedside (a Foley catheter). This is also painless and will drain your bladder until you are able to go to the bathroom by yourself. Most likely, you will also have oxygen prongs or a facemask for oxygen.

Despite the IVs and catheters, the nurse will get you up out of bed the first day following your surgery. This is very important to prevent post-op complications, such as blood clots and lung problems. A lung that is not breathing normally is very susceptible to accumulation of secretions, which in turn leads to accumulation of bacteria and pneumonia. In addition, the nurse or respiratory therapist will give you lung exercises to do to prevent this complication. It is important to have adequate pain control so that you feel like doing these exercises, so be sure to ask for and use pain medications as necessary.

You will not be allowed to eat or drink until the doctors are sure your stomach and intestines have woken up following the surgery. Typically, a patient's gastrointestinal (GI) tract tends to stop working for several days following a general anesthesia. When you start passing gas from below, you will be allowed to drink clear liquids. Your diet will advance as your stomach and small intestine become more active.

The most common complication following lung surgery is infection—usually a lung infection, often from not breathing deeply and/or clearing secretions out of the lungs. Other unlikely complications are bleeding, infections of the incision site, and post-operative heart problems, such as congestive heart failure or an irregular heart rhythm.

Make sure that you have adequate pain medications to take home. It is not uncommon for surgeons to underestimate post-op pain. Patients are often sent home with a small supply of pain medication when, in reality, many will need to take some medications for a month or longer. If your doctor does not want to give you a large supply, make sure you know how to contact him or her for refills.

**Mortality**

The number of people who die of a disease.

Healthy lifestyle behaviors post-surgery, including regular exercise, weight control, and healthy nutrition, have the potential to greatly reduce cancer treatment–associated morbidity and **mortality** in cancer survivors and can enhance quality of life. Recent research supports fitness as an important factor in long-term survival, decreasing the likelihood of surgery complications as well as reducing fatigue in cancer survivors. In fact, you should ask your healthcare providers about including exercise as part of your post-surgery rehabilitation therapy.

## 13. What is chemotherapy and how does it work?

Chemotherapy is a word for medications used to treat cancer. Unlike surgery and radiation, which are used to treat localized disease (in the lungs), chemotherapy is a systemic therapy used to treat disease that has spread to all parts of the body. Chemotherapy drugs are often administered intravenously (sometimes orally), and thus are absorbed into the blood. Since the blood flows to all parts of the body, in theory, cancer cells anywhere in the body would be exposed to the chemotherapy.

Most chemotherapy drugs work by interfering with the DNA of cancer cells. Because cancer cells divide rapidly and don't stop (uncontrolled growth), many chemotherapy drugs are specifically designed to target rapidly dividing cells. However, some normal cells in the body also grow rapidly—such as hair, the lining of the stomach, and blood cells—and chemotherapy can affect these cells as well, causing such side effects as hair loss, nausea (rarely vomiting), and susceptibility to infections. Ask your doctor about ways to prevent or reduce these side effects.

Chemotherapy sometimes consists of one drug, but more often it involves a combination of drugs called a **regimen**. Chemotherapy regimens combine drugs that have different mechanisms of action, or ways of attacking cancer cells, in order to increase their effectiveness and to prevent the cancer cells from developing resistance to chemotherapy. Your doctor will recommend possible chemotherapy regimens based on your type of lung cancer, your stage, the location of your disease, your general health, any previous treatments, the side effects of the drugs, and the goals of your treatment plan.

Above all, please note that the chemotherapy that is used to treat one type of cancer, such as breast cancer, colon cancer, or prostate cancer, is very different from the chemotherapy used to treat lung cancer, and the side effects will be much different. Although support groups are very helpful in supporting you during your treatment, the side effects that some of the patients with other cancers have experienced are likely to be very different than the side effects experienced by lung cancer patients. In addition, there are many different chemotherapy regimens for lung cancers. These have different side effects, too. For example, some are more likely to

**Regimen**
Specific chemotherapy treatment plan involving the drugs, doses, and frequency of administration.

**TREATMENT OPTIONS**

*35*

cause hair loss than others. Please talk to your doctor and/or nurse to get a realistic view of what you are likely to experience.

## 14. What can I expect during chemotherapy? What are the common side effects of chemotherapy?

The typical chemotherapy session begins with a standard blood test called a **complete blood count** (**CBC**). Because chemotherapy can lower your blood counts, your oncologist wants to be sure that your blood counts are high enough so that you are able to receive chemotherapy safely. You can ask your nurse or **phlebotomist** to use a small needle for your blood draw, which will minimize the discomfort caused when the needle is inserted into your vein.

The process of delivering IV chemotherapy is called an infusion. The most common IV method uses a thin needle or catheter (tiny plastic tube) that is inserted into a vein in your arm or hand. These IV needle sticks cause a bit more discomfort than a needle stick for a blood test because they require a slightly larger needle—the pain is a little sharper but just as fleeting. Some patients apply a numbing cream prior to needle sticks to make the process virtually painless. You might want to ask your oncologist or oncology nurse if this might be an option for you.

Once inserted, the needle or catheter is taped down to prevent it from moving and causing any pain. The chemotherapy drug(s)—and any pre-medications—are then dispensed from bags suspended from a metal IV pole. These liquids flow from the bags through a flexible tube

**Complete blood count (CBC)**

A blood test that counts the number of white blood cells, red blood cells, and platelets.

**Phlebotomist**

A technician trained to draw blood.

that feeds into the needle or catheter in your vein. An infusion pump is sometimes used to deliver a precise amount of medication over a set period of time.

You will receive your pre-medications (pre-meds) first. These will likely include fluids for hydration and anti-emetics to prevent nausea and vomiting. Your oncology nurse should clearly explain the pre-meds and chemo-therapy drugs you are getting. When the drugs begin to flow, you might feel a slight coldness or strange sensation at the IV site; however, the infusion pro-cess should be pain-free and uneventful. If you experience pain, burning, swelling, shortness of breath, or any other unusual reactions during your infusion, you should bring it to your nurse's attention immediately. Your nurse will check to see if the needle was inserted properly or perhaps adjust the flow of the medication to a more comfortable rate. There are other measures that can be taken to alleviate discomfort or other problems you might experience so you need to keep your nurse informed of your status.

The length of your infusion will depend on the number and amount of chemotherapy drugs you are receiving. Chemotherapy sessions can take 1 hour, several hours, or several days. Extended infusions might require a hospital stay, although these are unusual for most lung cancer regimens. For the duration of your infusion, it often helps to watch TV, read a book, listen to music, talk to a friend, sleep—do whatever relaxes you and makes the time go more quickly. You are unlikely to experience any side effects during the infusion. When your infusion is over, be sure your nurse has told you about any potential side effects, what to do if you experience them, and under what circumstances you should call your doctor's office. If your nurse tells you that you could experience nausea, don't leave the office without a prescription for medications to prevent nausea, and be sure you know how to use them.

In some instances, chemotherapy can be administered outside an office or hospital setting. For example, oral chemotherapies—in pill, capsule, or liquid form—can be taken by patients at home. Portable infusion pumps allow some IV chemotherapies to be delivered at home as patients go about their usual activities.

## Common Side Effects

The particular side effects that you experience will depend on which chemotherapy drugs you receive and your individual response. You should ask your oncologist or oncology nurse for information on the common side effects associated with your chemotherapy regimen. You need to be aware of how to manage the common effects and under what circumstances you should call your oncologist. Some patients find it helpful to keep a journal during chemotherapy treatment to record the dates, times, and duration of symptoms, along with descriptive information. The more accurate you can be in reporting your symptoms to your oncologist, the better care you will receive.

Although there are numerous side effects associated with chemotherapy, it is important to remember that no one gets all of them. In fact, most patients experience relatively few side effects. Common chemotherapy side effects include:

- Fatigue. Fatigue is one of the most commons side effects of chemotherapy, although for most patients, it is relatively mild. It tends to be at its worst for about 1 week following chemotherapy. Many lung cancer patients are able to continue working, although many cut back to part time. If your fatigue is overwhelming, tell your doctor because there could be something else going on.

- Hair loss (**alopecia**). Please note that not all lung cancer chemotherapy drugs cause hair loss. Ask your doctor.
- Mild nausea and, rarely, vomiting.
- Drop in blood counts (white blood cells, red blood cells, or platelets). This is called **myelosuppression** and is a potentially serious side effect of chemotherapy.

Less common effects include:

- Infection
- Loss of appetite
- Peripheral neuropathy (numbness and tingling of the hands and feet)
- Allergic reactions
- Sexual effects: desire, fertility, hormonal balance
- Oral effects: sore mouth and gums, changes in taste
- Gastrointestinal effects: diarrhea and constipation

## 15. What is targeted therapy? What are the common side effects of targeted therapies?

In order to understand what targeted therapies are, you need to understand a bit about the biology of a cell. Basically, everything a cell does—grow, divide, carry oxygen, absorb nutrients, pump blood, etc.—is dictated by the **DNA** of the cell. DNA is located in the **nucleus** of the cell (the center of the cell, wrapped in a membrane) and is packed together in 46 pieces called chromosomes. Chromosomes are made up of thousands of smaller units called "**genes**," each of which regulates a particular function (e.g., brown hair, blue eyes, etc.). If the DNA gets

**TREATMENT OPTIONS**

**Alopecia**
Hair loss.

**Myelosuppression**
A decrease in the production of blood cells.

**DNA**
The "brains" of a cell, which resides in the nucleus. In people, it exists as 46 "pieces," or chromosomes, half of which we get from our mothers, and half of which we get from our fathers.

**Nucleus**
The area of a cell where the DNA resides.

**Genes**
Segments of the chromosomes which direct the work the cell is supposed to do. For example, some genes will determine how tall a person is. Others may determine whether a person's eyes are blue or brown.

**Mutation**

Damage in the DNA. Depending on the mutation and where it is located, it may result in cancer. Cancer-causing mutations are often due to carcinogens (cancer causing substances) such as substances found in the diet or cigarette smoke. Some mutations may be inherited (usually not in lung cancer). There are many different types of mutations (deletions, insertions, amplifications, translocations, gene rearrangements, etc.).

**Driver mutation**

A mutation found in the DNA of cancer cells which causes, or drives, normal cells to become cancerous.

**Targeted Therapy**

A term for drugs which target specific mutations in cancer cells.

**Tyrosine Kinase Inhibitors (TKIs)**

Drugs which block a chemical reaction called tyrosine kinase. Most targeted therapies work by inhibiting this chemical reaction which is activated by a driver mutation.

damaged in some way, it is called a **mutation**. (There are many types of mutations: deletions, insertions, amplifications, translocations, gene rearrangements, etc.) There are many ways the DNA can get damaged; in lung cancer, the most common way is by the cancer-producing substances in cigarette smoke.

Scientists have started to learn about the different mutations that cause lung cancer. In some cases, it takes many mutations working together to cause cancer. Some mutations make a person more *susceptible* to getting cancer, but don't actually cause the cancer themselves. (In this case, your DNA needs a *second* mutation.) Some mutations don't do any harm at all. Others actually make things *better* (this is how we evolve)—for example, make us run faster, grow taller, be smarter, etc. However, some mutations *cause* cancer directly (e.g., no mutation, no cancer). These mutations are sometimes called ***driver* mutations**, because one mutation is all it takes to make a normal cell turn cancerous.

Scientists have also started to develop drugs which will block the action of these driver mutations. Since these mutations are only found in cancer cells, and these drugs specifically target the mutation, they are sometimes called ***targeted therapies***. In general, these drugs try to stop or inhibit the abnormal chemical reactions, sometimes called pathways, which are caused by the mutation in the cancer cell. Many of them inhibit a pathway which involves a substance called tyrosine kinase, so they are also sometimes called ***tyrosine kinase inhibitors***, or **TKIs**.

The most common driver mutation that causes non-small cell lung cancer is called **K-ras**. Unfortunately, scientists have not found a drug which can turn off K-ras, so sometimes people call it a "non-actionable" mutation, meaning that at this point we do not have a drug to block it. Other common mutations are found in the **Epidermal Growth Factor Receptor (EGFR)** gene or ALK gene. These are sometimes called "actionable" driver mutations because we can do something about these mutations—we have drugs which will block them.

It is estimated that between one-half to two-thirds of lung cancer patients have some type of driver mutation. They tend to occur primarily in patients with adenocarcinoma of the lung, although scientists are starting to identify some which cause squamous cell cancer and small cell lung cancer. Although K-ras is relatively common—it occurs in approximately one-fourth of patients with adenocarcinoma of the lung (see Question 3)—many of them are relatively rare. Some have only been found in less than 1% of lung cancer patients.

At the time of this printing, only three mutations have drugs approved by the FDA—EGFR, ALK, and ROS1. However, almost certainly more will be approved soon. Many drug companies are trying to make better drugs than the ones that were originally approved, or ones with less side effects. Sometimes these drugs are called "second generation" TKIs or "third generation" TKIs.

In some instances, a mutation can be found in more than one type of cancer—for example, a mutation in a gene called BRAF is common in melanoma, but also occasionally found in non-small cell lung cancer. There are several drugs approved by the FDA for patients with melanoma whose tumors have a BRAF mutation, but they are not yet approved for patients whose lung cancers have a BRAF mutation. Some oncologists will prescribe a BRAF drug approved for melanoma for a lung cancer patient with BRAF anyway. If one counts

**K-ras**

The most common form of mutation found in adenocarcinoma; at this point, no drugs have been developed to target it.

**ALK "Mutation"**

The ALK gene combines with another gene (i.e. the EML-4 gene). The resulting protein can cause cancer cells to grow and divide.

**Epidermal Growth Factor (EGF)**

A protein made by cancer cells that causes cancer cells around them to grow and divide.

**Epidermal Growth Factor Receptor (EGFR)**

The receptor on the surface of the cancer cell to which EGF binds. Once EGF binds to its receptor, a chemical reaction starts involving tyrosine kinase which causes the cell to grow and divide uncontrollably.

these types of mutations (drugs approved in one type of cancer but not lung cancer), then the number of "actionable" mutations goes up to about eight at the time of this printing. (The reason they have not been approved for lung cancer by the FDA is that the mutations are so rare in lung cancer that it takes a long time to study them and make sure they are active in lung cancer.)

Many people who have a targetable mutation and get treated with the appropriate drug can have dramatic and long-lasting responses. However, most of these drugs do not work forever—they do not cure patients, and at some point, the cancer starts to grow again. However, scientists are also starting to learn why the tumor becomes "resistant" to these drugs—and in many cases, it is because the tumor has developed a *second* mutation. And yes—scientists are already starting to develop drugs which target these resistance mutations as well.

**Actionable mutation**

A mutation for which there are drugs; for example, a mutation which can be acted upon by prescribing a targeted therapy.

**Sequencing**

A way of looking at the DNA of the genes to find out if they are normal or not.

**Fluorescent In-Situ Hybridization (FISH)**

A method of examining a tumor for a type of mutation called a fusion protein.

So how does one find out if one's tumor has an **actionable mutation**? Your doctor will send off a piece of your tumor (often from your original biopsy or surgery) to a special laboratory to have it *sequenced*. **Sequencing** is a way of looking at the DNA of the genes to find out if they are normal or not. Other mutations, such as ALK, are studied by techniques known as *immunohistochemistry*, or *IHC*, or *fluorescent in-situ hybridization*, or *FISH*. Some oncologists will just order three mutations to be sequenced (EGFR, ALK, and ROS1), since these mutations have drugs specifically approved by the FDA for lung cancer. Others will just order testing for the genes which are "actionable"—genes for which there are drugs approved, even if the drugs are approved for other types of cancers. Others will order *all* the DNA to be sequenced, even if we don't know if some of the mutations that are found cause cancer, or even if we don't have any drugs available for them, like K-ras. Ask your doctor which mutations he or she will test for.

Other points to note:

- The mutations that cause lung cancer are only found in lung cancer cells, and not in normal cells. They are also not found in sperm or egg cells, and thus they are not inheritable—*they cannot be passed down from generation to generation.*

- Also, lung cancer is *not* contagious—these mutations are not spread by breathing, sneezing, coughing, etc.

- With the exception of K-ras, these mutations tend to be found more often in people who have never smoked, although they certainly can be found in smokers or former smokers. Also, the majority of mutations we know about occur in patients with adenocarcinoma, although scientists are discovering some in squamous cell lung cancer and small cell lung cancer.

- Depending upon the type of mutation your tumor has, your doctor may order another biopsy if your tumor starts to grow again. This is to determine if it has developed a second mutation, as described above, for which there might be a drug.

- Biopsies are no fun, and there is a small chance of complications. For that reason, a blood test has been developed in which DNA shed from the tumor can be found. (Sometimes this is called a **"liquid biopsy,"** even though it is really not a biopsy at all—it's taking a tube of blood.) At the time of this writing, only one type of tumor mutation can be found in the blood—EGFR—and the test is not perfect. If an EGFR mutation is found in in your blood, the chances are very high it came from your tumor. However, if no EGFR mutations are found in your blood, it is possible that the tumor does have

**Liquid biopsy**
A blood test to determine if there is mutated DNA from a tumor in the blood.

an EGFR mutation, but did not shed enough DNA into the bloodstream to be detected. This is known as a "false negative," and your doctor may decide to order a tumor biopsy after all.

- Many companies are developing blood tests to look for other types of mutations, and others are developing tests to look for tumor mutations in the urine or saliva.

### Side effects

Since targeted therapies are very specific for cancer cells, they have less of an effect on normal cells. The most common side effects are different from the ones associated with chemotherapy (such as hair loss, nausea, or a drop in the blood count). Many people do not experience any side effects, and the ones they do experience are often mild. Although different drugs have different side effects, rash and diarrhea are two of the most common. The rash looks like acne and is typically scattered over the trunk and face. In some patients, it can be severe. If you develop a severe rash, talk to your doctor. He or she will probably prescribe skin creams or antibiotics and might reduce your dose. Other side effects include diarrhea, and occasionally, nausea or abdominal discomfort or fatigue. Be sure to ask your doctor which side effects are associated with the **targeted therapy** you are taking.

## 16. What are angiogenesis inhibitors, and what are the common side effects?

Tumors need a constant and growing blood supply to feed them, much like an advancing army needs a constant and growing supply of food and materials to sustain it. Formation of new blood vessels is sometimes called angiogenesis (angio = blood; genesis = new; angiogenesis = formation of new blood vessels), and drugs which stop this are called **angiogenesis inhibitors**. Blocking off this blood supply should, in theory, have two effects. It should choke off the cancer by stopping the flow of oxygen and nutrients to it, and it should stop the tumor from spreading through one of its usual highways—the bloodstream. (The other route cancer cells spread through is the lymphatics and lymph nodes.) **VEGF (vascular endothelial growth factor)** binds to its receptor on the surface of blood vessel cells and to the surface of tumor cells, not cancer cells. VEGF stimulates the blood vessel cells (endothelial cells) to grow, divide, and migrate into the tumor.

A common side effect of angiogenesis inhibitors is high blood pressure. Your doctor should be monitoring you for high blood pressure and, if need be, giving you blood pressure medications or adding to or changing the ones you are currently on. Another somewhat less common side effect is the loss of very small amounts of protein in the urine. Your physician could ask you to give periodic urine samples to check for this. A rare side effect of these drugs is coughing up blood, particularly in patients with squamous cell carcinoma. If this happens to you, notify your doctor at once because, very rarely, some patients with squamous cell carcinoma have died of this complication. *For that reason, patients with squamous cell carcinoma or patients who are coughing up blood should not be given these drugs.* Some doctors will withhold angiogenesis inhibitors from patients with large tumors that are located next to large blood vessels, although this has not been definitely shown to be a risk factor for bleeding.

**TREATMENT OPTIONS**

**Angiogenesis Inhibitors**
Drugs that prevent the formation of new blood vessels.

**VEGF (vascular endothelial growth factor)**
A family of growth factors, most often made by tumors, that causes blood vessel cells (vascular cells) to grow into the tumor.

## 17. What is immunotherapy and how does it work?

**Immunotherapy**

Drugs which boost the immune system and get the body's immune system to fight the cancer.

**Immunotherapy** is a way of treating cancer that differs from chemotherapy or targeted therapy. Chemotherapy works by killing actively dividing cells—hair cells, blood cells, cancer cells, etc. Some types of chemotherapy are given in pill form, but most are given IV. Targeted therapies are drugs which target specific mutations which are making the cancer cell grow, and are usually given orally (see Question 15). Immunotherapies are drugs which "boost" your immune system so it can kill the cancer, and are almost always given IV.

The immune system is your body's defense against infections. It is made up of different types of white blood cells, each of which fights bacteria and viruses together in different ways. The first step in getting the immune system to fight bacteria or viruses is getting it to recognize that these germs are not "normal" parts of your body. They are coming from outside your body, and therefore are "foreign" to your body. One type of white blood cell that recognizes that these are foreign substances is called a **T-lymphocyte**, or **T-cell**. T-cells are one of the first steps in activating the immune system. Just like T-cells recognize bacteria or viruses as abnormal or "foreign," they can also recognize cancer cells as being abnormal. Once they do so, T-cells become activated and can alert the rest of the immune system to fight the cancer.

**T-lymphocytes (T cells)**

A type of white blood cell which is important in recognizing an abnormal substance, such as viruses, bacteria, or cancer cells, and then activating the rest of the immune system.

So what goes wrong? If cancer cells are present, why don't the T-cells recognize that they are there and tell the other types of white blood cells to attack? The problem arises because of a unique way your body

46

has of telling the immune system to turn off once an infection is conquered. Some cancer cells use this system to avoid detection. Normally, once the infection is conquered, your body turns off the T-cells so they will stop activating the rest of the immune system. Normal cells do this by making a substance called **PD-L1**. PD-L1 binds to a protein called **PD-1** on the surface of the T-cells. When PD-L1 binds to PD-1, it prevents the T cells from "seeing" the germs as foreign, thus "deactivating" the T-cell. If the T cells can't "see" the bacteria or viruses, they stop activating the rest of the immune system. This is the way your body stops the immune system once an infection is conquered. If your T cells were not "turned off," they would continue to activate the immune system, eventually causing the immune system to over-react and attack normal parts of your body. (This is what happens in such **autoimmune diseases** as rheumatoid arthritis—the immune system attacks the joints because the suppression mechanism is not functioning properly.)

Some cancer cells evade the immune system by making their own PD-L1. Just like the compound produced by your normal cells, the cancer cells' PD-L1 binds to the PD-1 on the T-cells. This prevents the T-cells from "seeing" or recognizing the cancer cells, so that the T-cells are no longer able to "alert" or activate the rest of the immune system. It is as if the PD-L1 puts "blinders" on the T-cell—and if the T-cell doesn't know the cancer cell is there, it can't activate the rest of the immune system.

A number of drugs have been developed which prevent the PD-L1 made by cancer cells from binding to the PD-1 on T-cells. Some of these medicines bind to

**PD-L1**

A substance made by some normal cells to turn off the immune system. It works by binding to PD-1 on T cells. Some cancers cells also make PD-L1.

**PD1**

A substance found on T-cells which can bind to PD-L1. Once bound, the T-cell does not recognize the foreign intruder. It becomes inactivated, and in turn does not activate the rest of the immune system.

**Autoimmune diseases**

Diseases in which the body's immune system attack an organ.

*47*

PD-L1 and some bind to PD-1, but in either case, they prevent the PD-L1 from binding to the PD-1. This, in turn, prevents the T-cells from becoming "blinded." If the T-cell is not "blinded," it can recognize the cancer cell as being abnormal, and it can then activate the rest of the **white blood cells** to attack the cancer. These drugs are sometimes called "**checkpoint inhibitors**," since PD-L1 and PD-1 are also known as checkpoint proteins.

Why is it important to know all this about PD-L1 and PD-1? This is because your tumor can be tested for PD-L1, and the test might determine which of the many possible immunotherapies you can get. Testing is done by taking a small sample of your tumor (from a biopsy or surgery) and sending it to a lab to determine how much PD-L1 is present in the tumor or the surrounding tissues. Many studies have shown that patients whose tumor has a lot of PD-L1 are most likely to respond to immunotherapy, so the FDA has restricted the use of some of the drugs to patients whose tumors have "a little" or a "lot" of PD-L1. PD-L1 is tested by a special stain, and a "lot" of PD-L1 is often called greater than 50%, whereas some people consider a "little" PD-L1 expression as low as 1% or 5%. However, some patients whose tumors have no or very little PD-1 or PD-L1 have also responded. Clearly, one of the most important areas of immunotherapy research is trying to predict which patients are likely to respond. Ask your doctor if your tumor should be tested for PD-L1.

Immunotherapies are among the most exciting new treatments we have for cancer. These drugs can be very effective in some patients with non-small cell lung cancer. In about 20% of patients, it can shrink

**White blood cells (WBCs)**

One of the three major types of blood cells in the body. There are many types of WBCs, but their primary purpose is to conquer foreign "invaders," such as viruses, bacteria, and cancer cells.

**Checkpoint inhibitors**

A type of immunotherapy which works by getting T cells to recognize cancer cells.

the tumor for long periods of time—many months or even years.

However, there is a lot we don't know about them yet. Can they be combined with chemotherapy? Can they be combined with each other? Why do they work in some patients and not others? Why might they stop working after a period of time?

Also, because these drugs work so differently from chemo, they do not have the typical side effects of chemo. Many patients tolerate them very well, with almost no side effects. However, some patients do have side effects which result from the immune system getting boosted too much, causing what are known as "autoimmune diseases." (**Table 2**) Although these side effects are relatively rare, the immune system can attack the lungs, colon, liver, thyroid, or other glands or organs. Of these, the most common is hypothyroidism, which occurs in approximately 10% of patients. Hypothyroidism means that your thyroid gland stops making enough thyroid hormone, and usually can be controlled with thyroid replacement.

Fortunately, most of these side effects can resolve if the drug is temporarily stopped, and/or steroids are given. Unlike chemo, where the side effects are fairly predictable, these side effects can come at any time—immediately, weeks later, or even months after the immunotherapy is over. Because of the possibility of side effects, people who already have auto-immune diseases are not good candidates for these drugs. Your doctor should go over all the possible side effects with you carefully.

Immunotherapy inhibitors are often approved for different indications and certain stages of the disease

TREATMENT OPTIONS

(e.g., patients who are newly diagnosed or those who have failed chemotherapy or both); whether or not the tumor contains a little or a lot of PD-1/PD-L1 (or none at all), NSCLC vs SCLC, and whether they can be given alone or in combination with chemotherapy. Because the field is changing so fast, ask your doctor to get the most updated information as to which one might be right for you, and when.

Finally, if you have a targetable mutation (see Question 15), you should be treated with a targeted therapy *before* being treated with immunotherapy. This is because the chances of having a response to a targeted therapy—assuming you have the appropriate "target," or mutation—is greater than with immunotherapy.

**Table 2** Some possible side effects of immunotherapy*

| Parts of the body | Possible side effects and their names | Possible symptoms |
| --- | --- | --- |
| Thyroid | Hypothyroidism | Fatigue<br>Feeling cold<br>Weight gain |
| | Hyperthyroidism | Feeling warm all the time<br>Feeling jittery<br>Weight loss |
| Lungs | Inflammation of the lungs (pneumonitis) | Cough<br>Shortness of breath |
| Colon | Inflammation of the colon | Diarrhea |
| Liver | Inflammation of the liver | Decrease in appetite<br>Fatigue<br>Dark urine<br>Jaundice (development of a yellow tint of the skin or eyes) |
| Kidney | Inflammation of the kidney (nephritis) | Change in the amount of urine<br>Change in the color of the urine |
| Skin | | Rash |
| Other glands<br>Pituitary<br>Adrenal<br>glands | Hypophysitis<br>Adrenal insufficiency | Fatigue<br>Nausea<br>Headache<br>Electrolyte abnormalities<br>Dehydration |
| Eyes | Eye inflammation | Blurriness<br>Dry eyes<br>Pain<br>Light sensitivity |
| Neurologic | Guillain-Barre syndrome<br>Myasthenia gravis<br>Meningitis | Increasing weakness, particularly in the arms or legs |
| Infusion reactions | Reaction to the drug as it is being infused in | Fever<br>Chills |

*This is not a complete list of all the possible side effects of immunotherapy

TREATMENT OPTIONS

## 18. What is radiation therapy and how does it work? What are the common side effects of radiation therapy?

Radiation therapy (also sometimes referred to as radiotherapy, X-ray therapy, or irradiation) is the use of high-energy rays to stop cancer cells from growing or multiplying.

Radiation causes damage to the DNA, which is often permanent, causing cells to die. After cell death, the cellular remains must eventually disintegrate and be removed from the body. This dead cell removal can be quite slow and there could be a delay in the shrinkage of tumors receiving radiation even though all the cells are dead.

Radiation treatment is carefully planned to deliver as much radiation as possible to tumor cells while doing as little damage as possible to normal surrounding cells. Radiation is usually given in small doses over a long period of time to increase the effect on the tumor cells while providing intervals between treatments to allow injured normal tissues to recover, thus reducing the side effects of radiation.

**Rads**

A unit of absorbed radiation dose, defined as 1 rad = 0.01 Gy = 0.01 J/kg.

**Gray (Gy)**

The standard unit of absorbed ionizing-radiation dose, equivalent to one joule per kilogram.

**Centigray**

A unit of absorbed radiation dose equal to one hundredth (10−2) of a gray, or 1 rad.

The "dose" of radiation is measured in units called **rads** or **Gray** (**Gy**). One hundred rads equals one Gy or 100 **centigray**. The typical dose of radiation is about 6000 rads or 6000 centigray or 60 Gy. Rather than administer all 60 Gy in one treatment, the radiation is divided up into many treatments. The total dose of radiation and the number of treatments you will need will depend on the size, location, and type of your cancer.

Radiation delivered with "curative" intent usually consists of about 60 Gy given 2 Gy at a time, in 30 treatments or fractions, although your doctor will determine the best dose and number of fractions best for you. Treatments are typically given daily, although occasionally specific reasons require that treatment be given more frequently (twice a day) or less frequently (two to three times a week). Usually, radiation is given 5 days a week, Monday through Friday, over 6 weeks. Some data suggest that, in certain situations, giving the radiation therapy twice per day for a total of 12 days may be more effective than the standard schedule.

Radiation oncologists are also developing ways to give even higher doses of radiation (70 Gy or higher) without damaging surrounding tissue. When delivered to the brain, for example, it is sometimes given by a device called the "gamma knife" or the "cyber knife" (depending upon the type of device) or radiosurgery. When delivered elsewhere in the body, it is sometimes called stereotactic body radiation therapy, or SBRT.

## Common Side Effects

To get to the tumor, the beam of radiation has to pass through all the tissues in front of and behind the tumor, thereby generating side effects in these normal tissues. For example, radiation to a tumor in the chest must pass in through the skin, the normal lung, the tumor, and then go out through normal lung behind the tumor and then the skin. If the tumor is near the esophagus (or feeding tube) or spinal cord it might pass through a portion of these as well. Because of these side effects, radiation cannot be administered to the entire body; instead, it must be limited to the areas of tumor. The amount of radiation that any one area of the body can tolerate varies. Normal tissues that are extremely sensitive to the effects of radiation, and thus don't tolerate it well, include organs within the abdomen and the spinal cord.

The side effects of radiation relate to the amount and nature of normal tissues through which the beam of radiation must pass, as well as to the total dose of radiation given. Therefore, side effects will vary from patient to patient depending upon each patient's treatment plan. In general, however, common side effects of high-dose (60 Gy, or 6000 rads) radiation on various body tissues are as follows:

- *Skin*. Radiation side effects to the skin can include a sunburn-like rash. For lung cancer patients, this is rarely a major problem.

**Pneumonitis**

Irritation of the lungs.

**Fibrosis**

Scarring.

- *Normal lungs*. Radiation can cause irritation of the lungs (**pneumonitis**), which can result in shortness of breath and cough. In some patients, this can result in permanent scarring of the lungs (**fibrosis**). Although these side effects are mild and well tolerated in most patients, in some patients with underlying poor lung function, the loss of breath is so significant that the patient could end up on oxygen permanently. Sometimes, the radiation oncologist will prescribe steroids if he or she thinks radiation pneumonitis or fibrosis is the cause of the breathing problem.

- *Esophagus*. The esophagus is the tube through which food travels from the mouth to the stomach. Because it passes through the very center of the chest, it often gets exposed to radiation and can become irritated. Irritation of the esophagus usually feels like a sore throat, which can sometimes be so bad that patients have a hard time swallowing solid foods. This is a temporary side effect that usually occurs 3 to 4 weeks into the radiation treatment and continues for about 2 weeks afterward. Rarely, this irritation can cause scarring or fibrosis of the esophagus, which can result in problems with food getting stuck. If this happens, the patient might need an upper endoscopy, in which a gastroenterologist looks down into the esophagus with a fiber-optic tube or an endoscope and then uses a balloon at the end of the endoscope to squeeze open the scar tissue and dilate the esophagus.

If the sore throat experienced during radiation therapy becomes too bad, many radiation therapists prescribe a liquid anesthetic that can numb the throat, making it easier to eat. During this period of time, do not worry about eating a balanced meal, meat, or solids. It is more important to stay hydrated and consume as many calories as you can, usually in the form of high-protein or calorie shakes, puddings, creamed soups, and the like.

Recent studies in NSCLC patients undergoing chemoradiation treatment found that radioprotectants might reduce treatment-related esophageal symptoms. Ask your doctor if a **radioprotectant** is available to you.

**Radioprotectant**
A medication that reduces certain side effects of radiation.

- *Heart.* It is rare to experience heart problems from radiation. The radiotherapist is usually able to direct the beam of radiation so that only small areas of the heart are exposed.

- *Spine.* The spinal cord is very sensitive to radiation and therefore cannot tolerate high doses. Indeed, this is often a factor that limits the amount of radiation that can be delivered because side effects from spinal radiation are usually permanent. Irritation of the spinal cord can cause back pain and, rarely, numbness, tingling, and weakness of one of the legs, which, in extremely rare cases, can lead to paralysis.

- *Fatigue.* Fatigue is one of the most common side effects of radiation therapy. It is important that you get enough rest during this period. While fatigue can last from 6 weeks to 12 months after your last radiation treatment, it usually gets better 1 to 2 weeks after the treatment is finished.

## 19. What is combined modality therapy for lung cancer? What are the advantages and disadvantages of this approach?

Combined modality therapy usually means receiving two or more types of treatment: a local treatment (such as radiotherapy or surgery) and systemic chemotherapy. This is usually recommended when a patient has Stage II or locally advanced (Stage III) disease. Combined modality therapy is recommended because such patients often have a high chance of recurrence—either locally (at the site of the original tumor) or distantly (somewhere else in the body). In the latter case, if the cancer comes back somewhere else in the body, it is not the fault of the surgeon—presumably some cancer cells must have spread (metastasized) before the operation. A local recurrence also does not mean that the surgeon did not do his or her job—it means that microscopic amounts of cancer cells, too small for the surgeon to see, were left behind. Therefore, two types of treatment are needed: therapy aimed at the tumor itself (surgery or radiation) and therapy aimed at cancer cells that might have already escaped (chemotherapy or targeted therapy).

The subject of combined modality treatment, and how to administer it, is one of the biggest areas of controversy among lung oncologists. When should the doctor give the chemo? Before radiation or surgery? After? Which type of local treatment should you have—radiation or surgery? Both? Should the chemotherapy be given at the same time as the radiation? Which chemotherapy is best? Because medical knowledge regarding combination therapy is evolving, you should discuss the pros and cons of each of these approaches with your doctor.

One of the potential disadvantages of combined modality therapy is enhanced side effects.

- If high-dose radiation (60 Gy, or 6000 rads) is given before surgery, the normal tissues become so affected that the body has a hard time healing, and patients can have problems with wounds breaking apart inside the chest. Lower doses of radiation (45 Gy, or 4500 rads) are better tolerated preoperatively.

- Chemotherapy given concurrently (at the same time) with radiation instead of sequentially (one after the other), in particular, can have more side effects. Patients tend to experience many more problems with fatigue, sore throat, and swallowing. In addition, they are more likely to suffer from radiation pneumonitis and fibrosis (see Question 18). Nevertheless, because there is a survival advantage when the treatment is given this way, it is often recommended, particularly for patients with good performance status.

## 20. What are clinical trials?

Clinical trials are research studies involving people (as opposed to preclinical studies which could involve animals). Through clinical trials, scientists learn how to fight cancer. There are many types of clinical trials (prevention, screening, treatment, quality of life) and questions that scientists can address by means of a clinical trial. The clinical trials process is designed to encourage the development of new drugs for cancer while protecting the volunteers who participate in the trials.

Participating in a clinical trial can sound scary. However, this is the only way any progress is made in the

TREATMENT OPTIONS

treatment of cancer. All drugs that we now have to treat cancer were developed through clinical trials, in which patients such as you participated. There are many reasons for participating in a clinical trial, but even if you do not benefit directly, the knowledge gained from your participation will help future lung cancer patients. The clinical trials process for a new cancer drug begins with an application by the study sponsor to the Food and Drug Administration (FDA) to conduct a clinical trial. The FDA is the U.S. government agency that approves new treatments for marketing and sale to the public. It provides oversight and approval for new drugs, new devices, new types of treatments, and new uses for established drugs, devices, and treatments. For most cancer trials, the study sponsor is either a pharmaceutical company, the National Cancer Institute, or one of its associated trial groups, such as the Eastern Cooperative Oncology Group (ECOG), the Southwest Cooperative Oncology Group (SWOG), and ALLIANCE.

The study sponsor must demonstrate that testing of the drug in laboratory studies (in vitro studies, meaning in a Petrie dish or flask) and in animal studies (in vivo studies) showed promise with a reasonable expectation of safety in humans. After the investigational new drug (IND) application is approved, an investigational drug will usually undergo three phases of testing before it is eligible for final FDA approval:

- Phase I trials are designed to test the *safety* of the new drug. They usually involve a small number of patients (usually fewer than 50) who are given the drug in gradually increasing amounts to assess side effects and establish the most appropriate dose and schedule.

- Phase II trials determine how *effective* the drug is for treating a specific cancer. Phase II trials are usually conducted in larger groups of people (anywhere from 25 to 200). If the drug looks like it might have activity in a certain tumor type, then a Phase III trial is conducted.

- Phase III trials are designed to test whether a new drug is better than the standard treatment for a specific cancer. Both the effectiveness of the drug and the amount and extent of side effects are compared. The number of people participating in Phase III trials can range from hundreds to thousands and typically involve dozens of hospitals in the United States and sometimes worldwide.

Phase III trials frequently employ a trial design called a **randomized controlled trial** (**RCT**). In an RCT, the trial participants are randomly assigned (by chance, like the flip of a coin, although the randomization process is usually performed by a computer) to the treatment (experimental) group or the control (standard of care) group. You might hear these groups referred to as **arms**. The experimental arm receives the new treatment alone or the new treatment combined with standard treatment. The control arm receives the standard treatment. Assignment to one arm or another is not based on any medical information; it is random. Some trials are double-blinded, which means that neither the patients nor the doctors know who is in the experimental group and who is in the control group.

Randomization, control, and blinding are all scientific methods used to ensure that the trial results will not be

**Randomized controlled trial (RCT)**

A research study in which the participants are assigned by chance (using a computer) to separate groups that compare different treatments; a method used to prevent bias in research.

**Arm of a clinical study**

Treatment group to which a patient is assigned in a randomized clinical trial.

biased in favor of one outcome or another. If clinical trials were not randomized, physicians might tend to refer all of one type of patient or another to a particular arm of the study. For example, if the medical oncologist thinks a drug is particularly promising but is worried about side effects, given the option, he or she might decide to enter only the youngest patients into the investigational arm of the study and enter the older patients into the control arm, thereby possibly biasing the results.

**Placebo**

An inactive substance (e.g., sugar pill). Placebos alone are rarely used in cancer trials.

One type of trial design that concerns many patients is a **placebo**-controlled trial. A placebo is a dummy or inactive substance (like a sugar pill) that is given to individuals in the control arm of certain trials. Some cancer patients avoid clinical trials for fear of getting a placebo. This fear is unfounded. *It is extremely rare that a placebo-only arm is used in a cancer treatment trial.* It is unethical to treat patients with a placebo when effective care is available, even if it is in the context of testing a promising new drug. The only circumstances in which a placebo-only arm is used in a treatment trial is if the standard of care for that type and stage of cancer is no treatment at all or in an RCT in which the two arms are standard chemo plus study drug or standard chemo plus placebo. In either case, both arms get standard chemo. *Your doctor will tell you if a study involves a placebo*, but you should ask in any case.

# PART FOUR

# Coping with the Symptoms of Lung Cancer

## 21. Can my shortness of breath be controlled?

There are many causes of shortness of breath, and how to manage it will depend upon the cause. For example, if the shortness of breath is due to a pleural or pericardial effusion, the fluid can be removed to restore breathing capacity (see Question 24). Shortness of breath caused by emphysema or COPD can be managed with inhalers and antibiotics, and pneumonia with antibiotics.

There are several ways to relieve shortness of breath if it is due to the tumor blocking an airway. Radiation is often used to reduce the tumor, thereby relieving the obstruction or blockage. If the patient has already had maximal radiation, a **stent** can sometimes be placed. A stent is a device that looks similar to a hollow tube, which is inserted via bronchoscopy into the airway that is being blocked or crushed by the tumor. Other ways of relieving the obstruction include **brachytherapy**. Brachytherapy is a method of delivering a seed of a radioactive agent into the tumor that is blocking the airway.

Sometimes shortness of breath cannot be controlled using these methods. In these cases, the patient's shortness of breath symptoms can be managed with:

- *Oxygen.* Portable oxygen carriers are available to allow patients to be mobile.

- *Pain reliever medications* can reduce the uncomfortable sensation of breathlessness, so, although a person's body is not getting enough oxygen, the brain does not interpret it this way.

- *An anti-anxiety medication* will also help to relieve your feelings of breathlessness.

**Stent**

A hollow tube that can be inserted via bronchoscopy into the airway to prevent it from being blocked or crushed by the tumor.

**Brachytherapy**

Internal radiation therapy that involves placing seeds of radioactive material near or in the tumor.

## 22. Could I be depressed?

Depression is a common condition in lung cancer patients. Although patients who have a history of depression are most susceptible, many people who have never before experienced psychiatric problems could develop depression following a lung cancer diagnosis. Even though it is normal and natural to feel sad and down about the diagnosis, sometimes the feelings of sadness become so overwhelming that they take on a life of their own and become a problem in and of themselves. Patients can become so discouraged, hopeless, or full of despair that they are unable to enjoy their family or the little things in life. If you find yourself sitting at home all the time, no longer interested in your usual activities or in getting out of the house, withdrawing from your family, spending all your time in bed, and so on, you could be depressed. The good news is that most depression is treatable—and with medications that are usually well tolerated with minimal side effects. The bad news is that it frequently goes undiagnosed.

Several factors complicate the process of diagnosing depression in cancer patients. For example, many of the symptoms of depression (such as changes in eating and sleeping habits) are also symptoms associated with cancer and its treatment. Also, patients often do not openly share emotional symptoms—a major component of the depression diagnosis—with their doctors. If you think you might be depressed, it is very important that you discuss this possibility with your doctor. If your doctor does diagnose depression, he or she can treat you or refer you to a psychiatrist for further evaluation and treatment. Most frequently, cancer patients have reactive depression. Reactive depression is of limited duration and can be helped with counseling. Major depression is more severe and long lasting, and treatment most often includes medication, such as antidepressants. When depression is treated effectively, patients experience relief from distressing symptoms and are better able to cope with their cancer and the demands of cancer treatment. Recognizing the signs of depression early will help to quickly diagnose and successfully treat it.

Sometimes patients are unwilling to undergo treatment for depression, thinking that it represents a sign of weakness and that they should be able to control their feelings. Nothing could be further from the truth. When you are hungry, you cannot trick your mind into thinking you are not. When you have to go to the bathroom, you cannot trick your mind into thinking you do not. If you are depressed, why would you be able to trick your mind into thinking that you are not?

## 23. What can I do to relieve my pain?

First and most importantly, talk to your doctor. He or she cannot know you are in pain unless you speak up. Advocate for yourself. If one medication is not effective in relieving your pain or is causing a lot of side effects, tell your doctor. Do not wait until your next appointment—give the office a call. If they do not call back within a reasonable period of time, call again. You deserve to have relief from pain, and your doctor and nurse would agree with you if you let them know.

Everyone feels pain differently. Your doctor and nurse will often ask you to rate the pain on a scale of 1 to 10, with 0 being no pain and 10 being very severe pain.

Some patients agonize over this question, struggling with the difference between a four and a five, and they should not. There is no wrong or right answer, and your nurse or doctor will not quiz you regarding fine differences. This pain scale is simply a general way to determine whether your pain is getting better or worse.

There are many medications for pain. Typically, physicians manage mild pain with non-opioid medications, such as acetaminophen or nonsteroidal anti-inflammatory drugs (NSAIDs). Some type of opioid is usually required for moderate pain. Severe pain might require stronger opioids. Sometimes patients with severe pain might need to be hospitalized for intravenous medication to quickly control the pain and to determine how much oral medication they will need as an outpatient.

There are two major types of pain pills—short-acting and long-acting. Short-acting pills typically last about 6 hours and are generally used for pain that is mild, occurs occasionally, or comes and goes. Long-acting pain pills build up to a low but steady level in the blood. They could take a day or two to build up to an effective level so don't expect them to work right away. Short-acting pills are used to treat the pain you have at the time; long-acting pain pills are used to prevent it from occurring (or if it does occur, to reduce its intensity).

Short-acting pain pills are taken on an as-needed basis. Since long-acting pain pills take a while to build up in the bloodstream, they must be taken on a very regular basis, whether you are having pain or not.

Many patients feel they shouldn't have to take pain pills. Not so! You will do much better in the long run if you conserve your strength to fight the cancer instead of the pain. Remember—you don't get brownie points for putting up with pain.

Unfortunately, misconceptions about pain medications can sometimes prevent patients from taking these drugs or even talking to their doctor about pain relief. Some common misconceptions include:

- *I'm afraid of getting addicted to opioids.*

  Don't be. Numerous studies have shown that cancer patients in pain do not get mentally addicted to these drugs. They do not exhibit drug-seeking behavior and are able to be weaned off the medications without difficulty once the cause of the pain is controlled.

- *I want to save opioids for when I really need them.*

  Don't. Numerous studies have also shown that patients do not become tolerant to these drugs—that is, they do not find themselves requiring more and more pain medications for the same level of pain.

- *OK, but I'll still try to get away with taking as few pills as possible.*

  Don't. These pain medications are much, much better at preventing pain than taking it away once it starts. These pain medications are designed to be taken on a regular basis, whether you are having pain at that time or not.

- *Won't opioids make me woozy and lightheaded?*

  They might, but these are side effects that usually go away with repeated treatments. If you have this problem, try starting at a lower dose and slowly working your way up to allow your body to get used to it. If this doesn't work, tell your doctor, and he or she will try a different preparation. Although it varies a lot, some people have more of one kind of side effect on one type of pill than they do with another.

- *I'm afraid to take opioids because they make me so constipated.*

  This is one of the major problems with these drugs. It is extremely important to try to prevent the constipation— it is much harder to correct constipation after it has already occurred. Talk to your nurse or doctor about the various types of medications recommended to prevent constipation. Typically, most patients start by taking a laxative or stool softener at the same time that they take their pain medications. If you become constipated, try adding milk of magnesia. If that does not work, ask your doctor about taking the same type of medications that are used in preparation for a colonoscopy.

When using these medications, it is important to know that this is an area where the art of medicine comes in. Everyone is different, so play around with the timing, amount, and combinations of these medications until you have a combination that works for you.

- *What are other side effects of opioids?*

  Another possible side effect is nausea. Like constipation, if it cannot be managed with medications, ask your doctor to switch you to another type of preparation. Itching is a relatively rare side effect that can also usually be managed with medication.

- *What is the maximum dose of opioids someone can take?*

  The short answer is, "There is no one maximal dose— it depends on the individual." The side effect that eventually limits the amount of these medications

**Respiratory depression**

Slowing of breathing.

one can take is **respiratory depression**—slowing of breathing. However, most people are able to tolerate very high doses of opioids as long as the dose is increased gradually. A dose that would have very severe side effects in a person who has never taken these drugs might not faze a person who has been on them a while. So, even though patients do not become immune to the pain-killing properties of these medications, with time, they often become tolerant of the side effects.

- *I hate taking pills, period.*

  That is understandable; however, this is a time when the benefits could be far greater than any risks or concerns you might have about a pill. If you have difficulty swallowing pills, you can ask your doctor about a "pain patch".

  The medication, called fentanyl, gets absorbed through the skin over a period of time so the patch needs to be changed every several days.

- *I'm afraid to take these medications after all the stuff I've read about in the newspapers.*

  Don't be. Opioids, when taken for the appropriate reasons by careful individuals, are not harmful or addicting and are true miracle drugs for relieving pain. They only become problematic or addicting when used inappropriately by people who are not in pain. When used appropriately, opioids can be very helpful for lung cancer patients.

- *I've tried all these medications. They don't seem to work, and I have too many side effects. I'm afraid nothing more can be done.*

  Not so. Many times pain medication can be much more effectively controlled if it is given continuously through an IV pump. This small device, about the size of a cassette tape recorder, can be easily carried around with you, allowing you to live at home and perform your usual activities.

If your doctor is not able to effectively manage your pain, ask for a referral to a pain specialist or a palliative care doctor. They are experts in dealing with the various pain medications. In addition, they could know whether an injection or nerve block might be helpful.

## 24. What are pleural or pericardial effusions and how are they managed?

A pleural effusion is a collection of fluid between the outside of the lung and the chest wall (the **pleural space**). The lung is covered with a thin membrane called the **visceral pleura**, and the inside of the chest wall is covered with a thin membrane called the **parietal pleura**. Normally, the outside of the lung is touching the chest wall, and the space between the visceral and parietal pleura is virtually nonexistent. However, if there are tumor cells on either the visceral pleura or the parietal pleura, they can become irritated and cause fluid formation.

**Pleural space**
The area between the outside of the lung and the inside of the chest wall.

**Visceral pleura**
A membrane surrounding the lung.

**Parietal pleura**
A membrane lining the chest wall.

Other conditions besides cancer can cause fluid accumulation in the pleural space, including congestive heart failure or pneumonia. To prove that the pleural effusion is indeed due to cancer, your doctor will sample some of the fluid so it can be examined under a microscope by the pathologist. This is typically done as an outpatient procedure by numbing the skin with a topical anesthetic and then inserting a small needle into the chest and draining out some of the fluid.

One of the reasons pleural effusion is significant for lung cancer patients (in addition to the breathing problems it can cause) is that it exists in a free-flowing space. For example, when you stand up, the fluid settles to the bottom of the lung. When you lie on your side, it flows to the side and layers out along the side. If you were to stand on your head, it would flow to the top of the lung. As it flows, it can spread any cancer cells that might be floating within it, thus seeding other areas of either the visceral or parietal pleura. Because the fluid spreads the cancer cells around so extensively, local therapy, such as surgery and radiation, is usually not possible.

In most people, accumulation of some fluid in this area is not a problem. Some people, however, can experience shortness of breath, particularly if the pleural effusion is quite large. When it gets large, patients could also experience an uncomfortable sensation of fullness or discomfort in the chest, as well as a cough.

**Thoracentesis**

A procedure that uses a needle to remove fluid from the space between the lung and the chest wall.

The pleural effusion can be removed in an outpatient procedure called a **thoracentesis** (see **Figure 2**). In this procedure, a needle is inserted in the back between two ribs. It is attached to a tube that drains the fluid into a bottle or bag. The procedure is relatively painless. The skin is numbed with a local or topical anesthetic before the needle is inserted, so you will feel the needle to numb the area. After that, most patients do not feel anything, with the possible exception of a cough or vague discomfort if a lot of fluid is removed. These effects are due to the lung re-expanding.

**Pleurodesis**

A procedure to prevent recurrence of pleural effusion by draining the fluid and inserting medication into the pleural space.

If the fluid keeps reaccumulating, your doctor might recommend a procedure called **pleurodesis**. Although there are several ways of doing this, the procedures are all based upon the principle of draining the lung very,

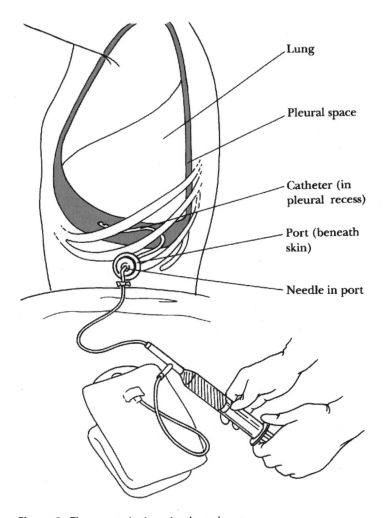

**Figure 2** Thoracentesis via an implanted port.

Reprinted from Yarbro CH, Frogge MH, Goodman M, and Groenwald SL. *Cancer Nursing: Principles and Practice, Sixth Edition.* Sudbury, MA: Jones and Bartlett Publishers, LLC, 2005.

very dry and then inserting some medication into the space where the fluid once was between the chest wall and lung. This medication is supposed to irritate the covering of the lung and the inside of the chest wall, which in turn is supposed to cause scar tissue (or fibrosis) to form between the two, thus serving as a type of glue to keep the surfaces stuck together. There are a number of different ways of doing this; the size of chest tube, the choice of medication, and whether the tube is inserted in the operating room or at the bedside will vary depending on local practices.

Regardless of exactly how the procedure is done, several points should be kept in mind. First, the procedure doesn't always work. This could be because it is impossible to get the pleural space dry enough, or because sometimes the lung will not re-expand. In addition, getting the pleural space as dry as possible often involves between 5 and 10 days in the hospital, usually with a chest tube inserted. For these reasons, most oncologists do not recommend pleurodesis unless it becomes clear that a patient is going to need repeated thoracentesis.

Sometimes, if a pleurodesis does not work, or if a patient chooses not to undergo the procedure, the surgeon can insert a small, semi-permanent tube called a **pleural catheter** into the pleural space that drains to the outside. Fluid can then be drained periodically as it accumulates. Once in place, the tube is painless and cannot be seen under clothing.

Just as the lungs are covered with a thin membrane called the visceral pleura, the heart is covered with a thin membrane called the **pericardium**. A **pericardial effusion** is fluid that accumulates between the heart and the pericardium. Sometimes, this fluid can hinder the heart from beating effectively, and it too might need to be drained in a manner similar to the pleural fluid.

**Pleural catheter**

Provides symptomatic relief of dyspnea related to recurrent pleural effusions.

**Pericardium**

A double-layered serous membrane that surrounds the heart.

**Pericardial effusion**

Accumulation of fluid inside the sac (pericardium) that surrounds the heart.

# PART FIVE

# *Living with Lung Cancer*

## 25. How should I change my diet following a lung cancer diagnosis? Should I take dietary supplements? Can diet affect my survival from lung cancer?

Many patients wonder whether changing their diet will improve their outcome. Frequently, patients will hear from friends and family that certain diets or foods will make a critical difference in their survival. You might hear, "Drink tons of green tea; it will cure your disease," or "Stay away from sugar; it will feed your tumor." Although some studies have shown that people who consume diets high in fruits and vegetables have a lower risk of developing lung cancer, there is no conclusive evidence that changing your diet after you have been diagnosed with cancer can affect long-term survival.

This does not mean there is no reason to pay attention to your diet. Eating a healthy diet is good for you and can certainly be beneficial when you are fighting a life-threatening disease. Eating affects how you feel, your energy level, and your overall health. The American Cancer Society's nutrition recommendations include: 1) Eat five or more servings of fruits and vegetables each day; 2) choose whole grains over processed (refined) grains and sugars; 3) limit consumption of red meats, particularly those that are high in fat and are processed; and 4) limit consumption of alcoholic beverages, if you drink at all. Of course, if you are suffering from cancer or treatment-induced weight loss, then you have special dietary needs and your doctor will advise you on what you can do to gain weight, or you can ask your doctor to refer you to a dietician or nutritionist.

There is also no definitive evidence that dietary supple-mentation can affect your lung cancer. If you do choose to take supplements, alert your doctor so that he or she can advise you as to whether the supplements might interfere with your cancer treatments. It is a good idea to take a multivitamin to ensure you are getting your minimum daily requirements of vitamins and minerals necessary for good health.

Most major medical centers have dieticians or nutrition-ists who specialize in helping patients with cancer. Ask your doctor or nurse.

## 26. If I smoke, is there any reason to quit? How can I quit smoking while dealing with the stress of lung cancer?

Yes, there are strong and compelling reasons for smokers to quit following a lung cancer diagnosis. The National Cancer Institute has found that cancer patients who continue to smoke could reduce the effectiveness of their treatment and increase the likelihood of a second cancer. There is also reason to believe that continued smoking could worsen the side effects of treatment, put you at increased risk for complications following lung surgery, and decrease your survival time. One study conducted in small cell lung cancer patients found that survival cor-related with smoking status. The patients who continued to smoke after their diagnosis had the poorest survival; the patients who quit at diagnosis fared better; and the patients who had quit on average 2.5 years prior to diag-nosis survived the longest.

Consider how the following health benefits of smoking cessation might affect you at this critical time in your life:

- Your circulation will improve.
- Your pulse rate and blood pressure, which are abnormally high while smoking, will return to normal.
- Your sense of taste and smell will return.
- Your breathing will become easier.
- Your risk of developing infections such as pneumonia (a common cause of death in people with lung cancer) is reduced.
- Your risk of developing other smoking-related diseases, including heart disease and other lung disease, is reduced.

It is never too late to quit. Even following your lung cancer diagnosis, smoking cessation will have a positive impact on your health, your quality of life and, possibly, your survival.

Your challenge is to motivate yourself to quit smoking during an extremely stressful time in your life. For some people this is easy—just hearing the words lung cancer is sufficient motivation. For others, the quitting process becomes even more difficult because smoking relieves the anxiety that comes with having lung cancer. Although quitting smoking is hard work (nicotine is very addicting) there are proven methods available to help you. The Surgeon General recommends **nicotine replacement therapy** (in patch, gum, inhaler, and nasal spray forms) as a treatment that increases long-term quit rates. In addition, there are also medications your doctor can prescribe to make it easier. These medications should start a week or two before you quit, to give them a chance to build up in your body. The effectiveness of these drugs is further increased with counseling,

**Nicotine replacement therapy**

Smoking cessation method that uses nicotine substitutes in various forms, including a patch, gum, inhaler, or nasal spray.

including behavior modification therapy, problem-solving or skills training, and social support. The more intense the counseling, the more likely you are to quit.

Your doctor can help you to find the combination of cessation methods that will work best for you and advise you on smoking cessation programs that are available in your community. Remember that you might have to make several attempts before you succeed—don't get discouraged. Keep trying and don't try to go it alone— seek support when you need it. For information on organizations, programs, and Internet resources to help you stop smoking, see the Appendix.

Not everyone who smokes and is diagnosed with lung cancer is able to quit smoking. Although there are definite health benefits, there are also understandable reasons why it is not possible for some patients with advanced lung cancer to quit. Scientists are learning that addiction to nicotine in some patients is due to chemical imbalances in the brain, making some patients more addicted than others. In those cases, it is important for the patient and the patient's family to let go of any guilt or anger over smoking. Conflict over smoking only serves to add additional stress on top of an already stressful existence. If you or your family cannot come to terms with your continued smoking, you should seek professional counseling to resolve this divisive issue.

## 27. What about returning to work? I am worried about being able to function at 100%. What are my rights?

Returning to work after time off for cancer treatment can be both physically and psychologically challenging.

You might have physical limitations as a result of your treatment, such as breathing problems and fatigue, which make full-time employment difficult. You might also worry about the reactions of your coworkers to your cancer and dread answering their questions about your health. The process of returning to work is different for everyone. Whether yours will be a smooth transition depends on a number of factors: the extent of your physical limitations, your comfort level in sharing information about your cancer with your coworkers, how supportive (and flexible) your employer is about your needs, your attitude toward your work, and the physical and emotional demands of your job.

Before you negotiate the terms of your return to work, it is important that you are aware of your rights and protections under both federal and state law. The Americans with Disabilities Act (ADA) prohibits discrimination by both public and private employers against qualified workers with disabilities or histories of disabilities. The Rehabilitation Act of 1973 ensures that federal employers or companies receiving federal funds cannot discriminate against cancer survivors (among others) in hiring practices, promotions, transfers, and layoffs. You could have additional employment protections depending upon the laws in your state.

Planning for your return to work can make a difference: Know your rights, consider how you will respond to questions from coworkers, and think ahead about what accommodations you might require on a short- or long-term basis so that you will be prepared to discuss your options with your employer. See the Appendix for resources that can assist you in determining your employment rights as a cancer survivor, provide information on how to ease your transition back to work, and direct you to resources you can turn to in the event that you suffer workplace discrimination.

## 28. What about follow-up care? How often should I be seen? What is my doctor looking for?

After you have completed treatment for your lung cancer, it is important that you receive regular follow-up care. Your doctor will want to see you to check for recurrence of your lung cancer, to manage any long-term effects from your cancer and its treatment, and to monitor for a second lung cancer or other primary cancer.

The American Society of Clinical Oncologists (ASCO) recommends the following follow-up schedule for asymptomatic (not currently showing symptoms of) lung cancer patients treated with curative intent: every 3 months during the first 2 years, every 6 months during years 3 through 5, and yearly thereafter. More frequent visits are warranted for patients with Stage III disease.

At each follow-up visit, your doctor will order certain blood tests, take a medical history, and perform a physical exam. X-rays and CT scans will be ordered regularly to monitor for recurrence in the lungs. Unfortunately, there are no standard recommendations for the frequency of these imaging studies, and practices among lung specialists vary widely. Although the brain and bone are common sites of metastasis in lung cancer, scans to detect metastatic disease (such as a brain MRI or a bone scan) are usually ordered only if symptoms are present.

The purpose of follow-up care, however, is to detect recurrence or disease at an early stage when it can be

**Palliative treatment**

Treatment given not with the intent to cure but with the intent to prolong survival and reduce symptoms from the tumor.

**Resection**

Surgical removal.

treated curatively or, if that is not possible, to begin **palliative treatment** in a timely manner. You will want to ask your doctor what symptoms you should be concerned about and under what circumstances you should report them.

Even though you are at high risk of recurrence during the first few years after your diagnosis, your risk declines as time goes on. You remain at increased risk, however, for a second, totally different primary lung cancer. Watching for a second lung cancer is important because **resection** of second primaries can be successful.

Although your main concern during your follow-up visits will undoubtedly be to make sure that your lung cancer has not recurred or that a second lung cancer has not developed, you should not hesitate to bring up other health issues that impact your quality of life. It is not unusual for patients to experience depression when their treatment stops, and you should discuss this with your doctor if you feel depressed or overly anxious and think you might benefit from counseling. Patients who have undergone chemotherapy, radiation, or surgery might experience long-term side effects that should be discussed on a regular basis so they can be properly addressed. Do not feel that your complaints are too minor to bring up during your follow-up visits. Your quality of life is important and your doctor should work with you to address these concerns.

# *Where Can I Find More Information?*

# *Lung Cancer Information*

### National Lung Cancer Partnership

Website: *www.NationalLungCancerPartnership.org*
Phone: (608) 833-7905
1 Point Place, Suite 200, Madison, WI 53719

The National Lung Cancer Partnership is the only national nonprofit lung cancer organization founded by physicians and researchers with lung cancer survivors and advocates. Its mission is to decrease deaths due to lung cancer and help patients live longer and better through research, awareness, and advocacy.

### American Society of Clinical Oncology (ASCO)

Website: *www.asco.org*
Phone: (571) 483-1300
2318 Mill Road, Suite 800, Alexandria, VA 22314

ASCO is a professional organization for cancer doctors. New findings in cancer research are presented each year at its annual conference. Conference abstracts are posted on the ASCO website.

### Cancer*Care*

Website: *www.lungcancer.org*
Phone: (800) 813-HOPE (4673)
275 Seventh Avenue, 22nd Floor, New York, NY 10001

A national nonprofit organization that provides free, professional support services to anyone affected by lung cancer. Services include counseling, education, financial assistance, and practical help. Information is available in Spanish.

### Cancer.net

Website: *www.cancer.net*

Oncologist-approved information for people with cancer, maintained by the American Society for Clinical Oncology (ASCO).

### Caring Ambassadors Lung Cancer Program

Website: *www.lungcancercap.org*
Phone: (503) 632-9032
P.O. Box 1748, Oregon City, OR 97045

Through state-of-the-art information, awareness efforts, advocacy, and support, the Caring Ambassadors Lung Cancer Program (CAP Lung Cancer) is firmly committed to bettering the lives of people living with lung cancer and their loved ones.

### National Cancer Institute (NCI)

Website: *www.cancer.gov*
Phone: (800) 4CANCER (422-6237)
(NCI's Cancer Information Service)
BG 9609 MSC 9760, 9609 Medical Center Drive,
Bethesda, MD 20892-9760

The NCI offers extensive up-to-date online and print information on lung cancer and its treatment, including clinical trials. Information is also available in Spanish.

### Lung Cancer Initiative of North Carolina

Website: *lungcancerinitiativenc.wordpress.com*
Phone: (919) 784-0410
Email: *HHooper@LungCancerInitiativeNC.org*
4000 Blue Ridge Road, Suite 170, Raleigh, NC 27612

## Print Publications

Henschke CI, McCarthy P, Wernick S. *Lung Cancer: Myths, Facts, Choices—and Hope.* New York: W. W. Norton; 2002.

Johnston L. *Lung Cancer: Making Sense of Diagnosis, Treatment, and Options.* Sebastopol, CA: O'Reilly & Associates; 2001.

*CURE: Cancer Updates, Research and Education.* Quarterly magazine that aims to explain scientific information to cancer patients. Print subscription is free to patients at *www.curetoday.com.*

## Caregivers and Home Care

### Family Caregiver Alliance

Website: *www.caregiver.org*
Phone: (415) 434-3388; toll-free: (800) 445-8106
785 Market Street, Suite 750, San Francisco, CA 94103

Caregiver resources include an online support group and an information clearinghouse. Information is also available in Spanish.

### National Family Caregivers Association (NFCA)

Website: *www.nfcacares.org*
Phone: (301) 942-6430; toll-free: (800) 896-3650
10400 Connecticut Avenue, Suite 500, Kensington, MD 20895-3944

NFCA provides education, information, support, and advocacy services for family caregivers.

### Guide for Cancer Supporters: Step-by-Step Ways to Help a Relative or Friend Fight Cancer (R.A. Bloch Cancer Foundation)

Website: *www.blochcancer.org*

### Print Publications

Houts PS, Bucher JA, eds. *Caregiving: A Step-by-Step Resource for Caring for the Person with Cancer at Home.* Atlanta, GA: American Cancer Society; 2000.

# Children

## Kids Konnected

Website: *www.kidskonnected.org*
Phone: (949) 582-5443; toll-free: (800) 899-2866
26071 Merit Circle, Suite 103, Laguna Hills, CA 92653

Nationwide organization that provides extensive support resources and programs for children who have a parent with cancer.

## Print Publications

Harpham WS. *When a Parent Has Cancer: A Guide to Caring for Your Children*, with companion book *Becky and the Worry Cup: A Children's Book about a Parent's Cancer*. New York: Perennial Currents; 2004.

# Clinical Trials Resources

There is no single resource for locating clinical trials for lung cancer. It makes sense to check repeatedly with all of the resources listed below because new trials are continually added. Clinical trials services are also emerging to help match patients to clinical trials. Some of these services can be useful for obtaining information and saving time, but it is important to read the company's privacy statement before using them and know whether the company is being paid for recruiting patients.

## ClinicalTrials.gov

Website: *www.ClinicalTrials.gov*

A resource provided by the U.S. National Library of Medicine with a database of privately and publicly funded clinical studies conducted around the world.

### NCI Clinical Trials

Website: *www.cancer.gov*
Phone: (800) 4CANCER

The National Cancer Institute (NCI) offers comprehensive information on understanding and finding clinical trials, including access to the NCI/PDQ Clinical Trials Database.

### NIH/NLM Clinical Trials

Website: *www.cancer.gov/clinicaltrials/search*

Clinical trials database service developed by the National Institutes of Health's National Library of Medicine.

### CenterWatch Clinical Trials Listing Service

Website: *www.centerwatch.com*

Listing of clinical trials, including trials sponsored by drug companies.

### Clinical Trials Resources

Website: *www.lungcanceronline.org*

In addition to linking to the major clinical trials resources listed above, LungCancerOnline provides links to NCI-designated cancer centers and hospitals with lung cancer programs that are likely to be conducting clinical trials in lung cancer. These sites can be contacted directly for information on available lung cancer trials. Links to some clinical trials services and directly to drug company trial information can also be found in LungCancerOnline's clinical trials section.

### NCI Clinical Trials and Insurance Coverage

Website: *www.cancer.gov*

Excellent in-depth guide to clinical trials' insurance issues.

## Print Publications

Finn R. *Cancer Clinical Trials: Experimental Treatments and How They Can Help You.* Sebastopol, CA: O'Reilly & Associates; 1999.

Mulay M. *Making the Decision: A Cancer Patient's Guide to Clinical Trials*. Sudbury, MA: Jones and Bartlett Publishers; 2002.

# Complementary and Alternative Medicine (CAM)

### American Academy of Medical Acupuncture

Website: *www.medicalacupuncture.org*
Phone: (310) 364-0193
1970 E. Grand Ave, Suite 330, El Segundo, California 90245

Professional site with articles on acupuncture, a list of frequently asked questions, and acupuncturist locator.

### National Center for Complementary and Alternative Medicine (NCCAM)

Website: *http://nccam.nih.gov/*

Offers information on complementary and alternative medicine therapies, including NCI/PDQ expert-reviewed fact sheets on individual therapies and dietary supplements.

### NCI Office of Cancer Complementary and Alternative Medicine (OCCAM)

Website: *http://cam.cancer.gov/*

Information clearinghouse supporting the NCI's CAM activities.

## Print Publications

American Cancer Society. *American Cancer Society's Guide to Complementary and Alternative Cancer Methods*. Atlanta, GA: American Cancer Society; 2000.

Kaptchuk TJ. *The Web That Has No Weaver: Understanding Chinese Medicine*. New York: McGraw-Hill; 2000.

# Diet and Nutrition

### American Institute for Cancer Research

Website: *www.aicr.org*
Phone: (202) 328-7744; toll-free: (800) 843-8114
1759 R Street, NW, Washington, DC 20009

Supports research on diet and nutrition in the prevention and treatment of cancer. Provides information to cancer patients on nutrition and cancer, including a compilation of healthy recipes. Maintains a nutrition hotline for questions relating to nutrition and health.

### Nutrition (American Cancer Society [ACS])

Website: *www.cancer.org* (Enter *Nutrition* in the search box.)

Nutrition resources include ACS guidelines on nutrition, dietary supplement information, nutrition message boards, and tips on low-fat cooking and choosing healthy ingredients.

# Drugs/Medications

### MedlinePlus: Drug Information

Website: *www.medlineplus.gov*
(Click on *Drugs & Supplements*.)

Database with information on thousands of prescription and over-the-counter medications. Maintained by the National Library of Medicine.

### Print Publications

Wilkes G. *Consumers Guide to Cancer Drugs*. Sudbury, MA: Jones and Bartlett Publishers; 2003.

# Employment, Insurance, Financial, and Legal Resources

### Americans with Disabilities Act
### (U.S. Department of Justice)

Website: *www.ada.gov*

Provides information and technical assistance related to the ADA.

### America's Health Insurance Plans (AHIP)

Website: *www.ahip.org*

Provides insurance guides for consumers. Topics include health insurance, managed care, disability income, and long-term care.

### Cancer Legal Resource Center

Website: *www.lls.edu/academics/centersprograms/
    cancerlegalresourcecenter/*
Phone: (213) 736-1031; toll-free: (866) THE-CLRC
919 Albany Street, Los Angeles, CA 90015

A joint program of the Disability Rights Legal Center and Loyola Law School. Provides free information and resources on cancer-related legal issues to survivors, caregivers, health-care professionals, employers, and others coping with cancer.

### Centers for Medicare and Medicaid Services (CMS)
*(Formerly the Health Care Financing Administration [HCFA])*
Website: *www.cms.hhs.gov*

The CMS is a federal agency within the U.S. Department of Health and Human Services that oversees administration of Medicare and Medicaid.

## Medicare

Website: *www.medicare.gov*
Phone: (800) MEDICARE

Federal health insurance program for people 65 years or older and some disabled people under 65 years.

## Medicaid

Website: *www.medicaid.gov*

Federal and state health assistance program for certain low-income people.

## Health Insurance Portability and Accountability Act (HIPAA)

Website: *www.hhs.gov/ocr/privacy/*

Insurance reform that might lower your chance of losing existing coverage, ease your ability to switch health plans, and/or help you buy coverage on your own if you lose your employer's plan and have no other coverage available.

## Family and Medical Leave Act (FMLA)

Website: *www.dol.gov/whd/fmla/*

U.S. Department of Labor website, providing information about the FMLA.

## Hill-Burton Program
## (Health Resources and Services Administration)

Website: *www.hrsa.gov*
(Enter *Hill-Burton Program* in the search box.)
Phone: (800) 638-0742; in Maryland: (800) 492-0359

Facilities that receive Hill-Burton funds from the government are required by law to provide free services to some people who cannot afford to pay. Information on Hill-Burton eligibility and facilities locations is available via phone or Internet.

## Patient Advocate Foundation

Website: *www.patientadvocate.org*
Phone: (800) 532-5274
421 Butler Farm Road, Hampton, VA 23666

Nonprofit organization helps patients to resolve insurance, debt, and job discrimination matters relative to their cancer diagnosis through case managers, doctors, and attorneys.

## Social Security Administration (SSA)

Website: *www.ssa.gov*
Phone: (800) 772-1213

Oversees two programs that pay benefits to people with disabilities:
- Social Security Disability Insurance—pays benefits to you and certain members of your family if you have worked long enough and paid Social Security taxes.
- Supplemental Security Income—supplements Social Security payments based on need.

## Veterans Health Administration

Website: *www.va.gov*
(Click on *Veteran Services*, then *Health Care*.)
Phone: (800) 827-1000; healthcare benefits: (877) 222-8387

Eligible veterans and their dependents could receive cancer treatment and care at a Veterans Administration Medical Center.

# Print Publications

Landry DS. *Be Prepared: The Complete Financial, Legal, and Practical Guide to Living with Cancer, HIV, and Other Life-Challenging Conditions.* New York: St. Martin's Press; 1998.

# Financial Assistance Programs

### Air Care Alliance

Website: *www.aircareall.org*
Phone: (888) 260-9707

Network of organizations willing to provide public benefit flights for health care.

### Finding Ways to Pay for Care
### (National Coalition for Cancer Survivorship)

Website: *www.canceradvocacy.org.*
(Select *Cancer Resources* and then *Cancer Survival Toolbox.*)

### Partnership for Prescription Assistance

Website: *www.pparx.org*

Coalition of drug companies and other groups to help qualifying patients get the medicines they need for free or very low cost through public and private programs.

# Hospice and End-of-Life Issues

### Growth House

Website: *www.growthhouse.org*

Extensive annotated directory to hospice and end-of-life resources. Organized by topic.

### Home Care Guide for Advanced Cancer
### (American College of Physicians)

Website: *www.acponline.org*

Guide for family and friends caring for advanced cancer patients who are living at home.

**Hospice Net**

Website: *www.hospicenet.org*

Provides comprehensive information to patients and families facing life-threatening illness. Extensive resources addressing end-of-life issues from both patient and caregiver perspectives.

## Patient Self-Advocacy Skills

**Cancer Survival Toolbox**
**(National Coalition for Cancer Survivorship)**

Website: *www.canceradvocacy.org*
(Select *Cancer Resources* and then *Cancer Survival Toolbox*.)

Topics include communication skills, finding information, solving problems, making decisions, negotiating, and standing up for your rights. (Also available as audiotapes at [877] 866-5748.)

**Questions to Ask Your Doctor**

Website: *www.cancer.net*
(Enter *Doctor Questions* in the search box.)

## Physician and Hospital Locators

**Finding the Best Lung Cancer Care**

Website: *www.lungcanceronline.org*

Provides links to databases of lung cancer specialists (e.g., oncologists, thoracic surgeons) maintained by professional organizations and a listing of medical institutions that offer multidisciplinary lung cancer programs, including NCI-designated cancer centers.

# *Prevention and Risk Assessment*

### Cancer Research and Prevention Foundation

Website: *www.preventcancer.org*
Phone: (703) 836-4412; toll-free: (800) 227-2732
1600 Duke Street, Suite 500, Alexandria, VA 22314

Offers information on prevention and early detection of cancer.

### Your Cancer Risk (Harvard School of Public Health)

Website: *www.diseaseriskindex.harvard.edu*
(Click on *Cancer.*)

Online assessment tool that estimates your lung cancer risk
and provides tips for prevention.

# *Research Resources and Reference*

### Dictionary of Cancer Terms (National Cancer Institute)

Website: *www.cancer.gov*

### Medscape

Website: *www.medscape.com*
(Enter *Lung Cancer* in the search box.)

Medscape is an excellent source for the latest news in lung
cancer research, including access to summaries of cancer
conferences. Aimed at healthcare professionals. Registration
required for free access to Medscape.

### PubMed: MEDLINE (National Library of Medicine)

Website: *www.pubmed.org*

Provides free online access to MEDLINE, a database of
more than 15 million citations to the medical literature.

## Print Publications

Laughlin EH. *Coming to Terms with Cancer: A Glossary of Cancer-Related Terms.* Atlanta, GA: American Cancer Society; 2002

# Smoking Cessation

### Quitnet

Website: *www.quitnet.com*

Comprehensive website for smoking cessation needs. Offers interactive personalized quitting tools, quitting guides, smoking cessation program locators, 24-hour online support/discussion, and links to smoking, tobacco, and cessation-related information and resources.

### Smokefree.gov

Website: *www.smokefree.gov*

Information and professional assistance for people trying to quit smoking. Resources include cessation guides, telephone quit lines, instant messaging service, and print publications. Sponsored by the National Cancer Institute, the Centers for Disease Control and Prevention, and the American Cancer Society.

# Support Services

### Association of Cancer Online Resources (ACOR)

Website: *www.acor.org* (Enter *Lung Cancer* in the search box.)

ACOR offers online support groups for cancer patients. Lung cancer lists include a general list (LUNG-ONC), lists for small cell lung cancer (LUNG-SCLC), lists for non-small cell lung cancer (LUNG-NSCLC), and lists for bronchioloalveolar carcinoma (LUNG-BAC). Also offers a wide variety of support groups for general and specific cancer- and treatment-related issues.

### Cancer*Care*

Website: *www.cancercare.org*
Phone: (212) 712-8400; toll-free: (800) 813-4673
275 Seventh Avenue, New York, NY 10001

Provides comprehensive support services and programs to people with cancer.

### National Lung Cancer Partnership

Website: *www.nationallungcancerpartnership.org*
Phone: (608) 833-7905
1 Point Place, Suite 200, Madison, WI 53719

Provides services under Living with Lung Cancer, such as educational materials, inspirational stories, blogs, and clinical trial information.

### Phone Buddy Program (Lung Cancer Alliance)

Website: *www.lungcanceralliance.org*
(Enter *Phone Buddy* in the search box.)
Phone: (800) 298-2436

Offers peer-to-peer telephone support. Matches lung cancer survivors or their caregivers and family members with individuals who have faced, or are facing, similar circumstances.

### R. A. Bloch National Cancer Foundation

Website: *www.blochcancer.org*
Phone: (816) 854-5050; toll-free: (800) 433-0464
4400 Main Street, Kansas City, MO 64111

Provides Bloch-authored cancer books free of charge, a multidisciplinary referral service, and patient-to-patient phone support.

**Vital Options International**

Website: *www.vitaloptions.org*
Phone: (818) 508-5657
4419 Coldwater Canyon Ave., Suite I, Studio City, CA
91604-1479

Produces "The Group Room," a weekly, syndicated radio call-in show (with simultaneous webcast) covering important and timely topics in cancer. Previous shows are archived for access on the website.

**Wellness Community**

Website: *www.thewellnesscommunity.org*
Phone: (202) 659-9709; toll-free: (800) 793-WELL
1050 17th Street NW, Suite 500, Washington, DC 20036

Provides educational programs and support groups for people with cancer and their families.

## Print Publications

Holland JC, Lewis S. *The Human Side of Cancer*. New York: Perennial Currents; 2001.

Schimmel SR, Fox B. *Cancer Talk: Voices of Hope and Endurance from "The Group Room," the World's Largest Cancer Support Group*. New York: Broadway Books; 1999.

St. John TM. *With Every Breath: A Lung Cancer Guidebook*. Vancouver, WA: The Lung Cancer Caring Ambassador's Program; 2005. Also available online at *www.lungcancerguidebook.org*.

# Symptoms, Side Effects, and Complications

## FATIGUE

### Cancer—Fatigue
### (Association of Cancer Online Resources)

Website: *www.acor.org*
(Enter *Cancer Fatigue* in the search box.)

Online discussion list covering cancer and treatment-related fatigue.

### National Cancer Institute

Website: *www.cancer.gov*
(Enter *Fatigue* in the search box.)
Phone: (800) 4CANCER

### American Cancer Society

Website: *www.cancer.org*
Phone: (800) ACS-2345

### NCI/PDQ Fatigue

Website: *www.cancer.gov*
(Enter *Fatigue* in the search box.)

Expert-reviewed information summary about cancer-related fatigue.

## Print Publications

Harpham WS. Resolving the frustration of fatigue. *A Cancer Journal for Clinicians*. 1999;49:178–189.

Outstanding article by a patient/physician which discusses cancer-related fatigue and how to deal with it.

# NAUSEA AND VOMITING

## NCI/PDQ Nausea and Vomiting

Website: *www.cancer.gov*
(Enter *Nausea* in the search box.)

Expert-reviewed information summary about nausea and vomiting related to cancer and its treatments.

# NUTRITIONAL PROBLEMS

## NCI/PDQ Nutrition

Website: *www.cancer.gov*
(Enter *Nutrition* in the search box.)

Expert-reviewed information summary about the causes and management of nutritional problems occurring in cancer patients.

# ORAL COMPLICATIONS

## NCI/PDQ Oral Complications of Chemotherapy and Head/Neck Radiation

Website: *www.cancer.gov*
(Enter *Oral Complications* in the search box.)

# PAIN

## NCI/PDQ Pain

Website: *www.cancer.gov*
(Enter *Pain* in the search box.)

Expert-reviewed information summary about cancer-related pain. Includes discussion of approaches to the management and treatment of cancer-associated pain.

## Print Publications

Abrahm JL. *A Physician's Guide to Pain and Symptom Management in Cancer Patients*, 2nd ed. Baltimore, MD: The Johns Hopkins University Press; 2005.

Aimed at healthcare professionals, this practical and comprehensive textbook is also an excellent resource for patients.

# PERIPHERAL NEUROPATHY

### The Neuropathy Association

Website: *www.neuropathy.org*
Phone: (212) 692-0662
60 East 42nd Street, Suite 942, New York, NY 10165

### Cancer—Neuropathy
### (Association of Cancer Online Resources)

Website: *www.acor.org*
(Enter *Cancer Neuropathy* in the search box.)

Online discussion group for patients dealing with neuropathy induced by cancer or its treatments.

## Print Publications

Almadrones LA, Arcot R. Patient guide to peripheral neuropathy. *Oncology Nursing Forum.* 1999;26(8):1359–1362.

# PLEURAL EFFUSION: SEXUAL EFFECTS

### Cancer—Fertility and Cancer—Sexuality
### (Association of Cancer Online Resources)

Website: *www.acor.org*
(Enter *Cancer Sexuality* in the search box.)

Online discussion lists about fertility and sexuality issues associated with cancer.

**NCI/PDQ Sexuality and Reproductive Issues**

Website: *www.cancer.gov*
(Enter *Sexuality* in the search box.)

Expert-reviewed information summary about factors that could affect fertility and sexual functioning in people who have cancer.

## Tests and Procedures

**Cancer Imaging (National Cancer Institute)**

Website: *www.cancer.gov*
(Enter *Cancer Imaging* in the search box.)

**Laboratory Tests (MEDLINEplus)**

Website: *www.nlm.nih.gov*

### Print Publications

Margolis S, ed. *The Johns Hopkins Consumer Guide to Medical Tests: What You Can Expect, How You Should Prepare, What Your Results Mean.* New York City, NY: Rebus, Inc.; 2001.

## Treatment Information and Guidelines

**NCI/PDQ Non-Small Cell Lung Cancer Treatment and Small Cell Lung Cancer Treatment**

Website: *www.cancer.gov*
(Enter *Lung Cancer* in the search box and then select the first suggested link.)

Expert-reviewed summaries about the treatment of NSCLC and SCLC.

**Chemotherapy and You (NIH/NCI)**

Website: *www.cancer.gov*
(Enter *Chemotherapy and You* in the search box.)

Also available in print by calling (800) 4CANCER.

**Radiation Therapy and You (NIH/NCI)**

Website: *www.cancer.gov*
(Enter *Radiation Therapy and You* in the search box.)

Also available in print by calling (800) 4CANCER.

**Surgery for Lung Cancer (CancerHelp UK)**

Website: *www.cancerhelp.org.uk*
(Enter *Surgery for Lung Cancer* in the search box.)

## *Living Well with Cancer*

**LT-SURVIVORS**
**(Association of Cancer Online Resources)**

Website: *www.acor.org*
(Enter *Long-term Survivors* in the search box.)

Forum for discussion of issues of concern to long-term cancer survivors.

**National Coalition for Cancer Survivorship (NCCS)**

Website: *www.canceradvocacy.org*
Phone: (301) 650-9127; toll-free: (877) NCCS-YES
1010 Wayne Avenue, Suite 770, Silver Spring, MD 20910

### Print Publications

Harpham WS. *After Cancer: A Guide to Your New Life.* New York: PerennialCurrents; 1995.

## *Women and People of Color*

### National Lung Cancer Partnership

Website: *www.nationallungcancerpartnership.org*
Phone: (608) 833-7905
1 Point Place, Suite 200, Madison, WI 53719

### Office of Minority Health

Website: *www.minorityhealth.hhs.gov*
Phone: (240) 453-2882
1101 Wootton Parkway, Suite 600, Rockville, MD 20852

### WomensHealth.gov

Website: *www.womenshealth.gov*
Phone: (202) 690-7650
200 Independence Avenue, SW, Washington, DC 20201

## A

**Actionable mutation**: A mutation for which there are drugs; for example, a mutation which can be acted upon by prescribing a targeted therapy.

**Adenocarcinoma**: A type of non-small cell lung cancer; a malignant tumor that arises from glandular tissue.

**Adenocarcinoma-in-situ (AIS)**: Formerly called bronchioloalveolar carcinoma, a subtype of adenocarcinoma sometimes found in non-smokers.

**ALK "Mutation"**: The ALK gene combines with another gene (i.e. the EML-4 gene). The resulting protein can cause cancer cells to grow and divide.

**Alopecia**: Hair loss.

**Alveoli**: Tiny air sacs that compose the lungs.

**Angiogenesis inhibitors**: Drugs that prevent the formation of new blood vessels.

**Antibodies**: Proteins found in the blood that detect and destroy invaders, like bacteria and viruses.

**Apoptosis**: Process by which normal cells die when they are injured; often referred to as programmed cell death.

**Arm of a clinical study**: Treatment group to which a patient is assigned in a randomized clinical trial.

**Autoimmune diseases**: Diseases in which the body's immune system attack an organ.

## B

**Benign**: Not cancerous; not life threatening.

**Biopsy**: Removal of tissue or fluid sample for microscopic examination.

**Brachytherapy**: Internal radiation therapy that involves placing seeds of radioactive material near or in the tumor.

**Bronchioloalveolar carcinoma (BAC)**: Now called adenocarcinoma-in-situ (AIS). A type of adenocarcinoma.

**Bronchoscope**: See Bronchoscopy.

**Bronchoscopy**: A procedure that involves inserting a flexible tube (bronchoscope) through the nose down into the lungs. Needles can be inserted through the bronchoscope to obtain biopsy samples.

## C

**Cells**: Microscopic units that make up the organs of the body.

**Centigray**: A unit of absorbed radiation dose equal to one hundredth (10–2) of a gray, or 1 rad.

**Checkpoint inhibitors**: A type of immunotherapy which works by getting T cells to recognize cancer cells.

**Chemotherapy**: The use of medicine to treat cancer; a whole-body or systemic treatment.

**Chronic obstructive pulmonary disease (COPD)**: Emphysema and chronic bronchitis are the two most common forms of COPD.

**Complete blood count (CBC)**: A blood test that counts the number of white blood cells, red blood cells, and platelets.

**Cytokines**: Proteins made by the cells that act on other cells to stimulate or inhibit their function.

## D

**DNA:** The "brains" of a cell, which resides in the nucleus. In people, it exists as 46 "pieces," or chromosomes, half of which we get from our mothers, and half of which we get from our fathers.

**Driver mutation**: A mutation found in the DNA of cancer cells which causes, or drives, normal cells to become cancerous.

## E

**Epidermal growth factor (EGF)**: A protein made by cancer cells that causes cancer cells around them to grow and divide.

**Epidermal growth factor (EGFR)**: The receptor on the sur-face of the cancer cell to which EGF binds.

**EML-4/ALK fusion protein**: An abnormal protein made when two genes combine (i.e., the EML-4 gene and the ALK gene). The resulting protein can cause cancer cells to grow and divide.

**Esophagus**: The tube through which food travels from the mouth to the stomach.

## F

**Fibrosis**: Scarring.

**Fluorescent In-Situ Hybridization (FISH)**: A method of examining a tumor for a type of mutation called a fusion protein.

## G

**Genes**: Segments of the chromosomes which direct the work the cell is supposed to do. For example, some genes will determine how tall a person is. Others may determine whether a person's eyes are blue or brown.

**Growth factors**: Substances that stimulate cells to grow; drugs that help the bone marrow recover from the effects of chemotherapy.

**Growth factor inhibitors**: Substances that inhibit the growth factors that stimulate cells to grow.

## H

**Hilar lymph nodes**: Lymph nodes located in the region where the bronchus meets the lung.

## I

**Incidence**: The number of new cases of a cancer (or any disease or event) in a defined population during a set period of time.

**Immunotherapy**: Drugs which boost the immune system and get the body's immune system to fight the cancer.

**Interventional radiologist**: A radiologist who uses X-rays and other imaging techniques to perform minimally invasive medical procedures.

**Intravenous**: In the vein.

## K

**K-ras**: The most common form of mutation found in adenocarcinoma; at this point, no drugs have been developed to target it.

## L

**Large cell carcinoma**: A type of non-small cell lung cancer.

**Ligand**: A molecule that binds to another chemical entity to form a larger complex.

**Liquid biopsy**: A blood test to determine if there is mutated DNA from a tumor in the blood.

**Lobectomy**: Surgical removal of a lobe of the lung.

**Lobes**: Clear anatomical divisions or extensions that can be determined without the use of a microscope (at the gross anatomy level). The right lung contains three lobes and the left contains two.

**Lymph node**: Small collections of white blood cells scattered throughout the body.

**Lymph node dissection**: Surgical removal of lymph nodes.

**Lymphatic system**: A vascular system that contains lymph nodes through which white blood cells flow; cancer can also spread through the lymphatic system.

# M

**Main stem bronchi**: The two main breathing tubes (right main stem bronchus and left main stem bron-chus) that branch off the trachea.

**Malignant**: Cancerous; cells that exhibit rapid, uncontrolled growth and can spread to other parts of the body.

**Mediastinal lymph nodes**: Lymph nodes located in the mediastinum, the area between the lungs.

**Mediastinoscopy**: A surgical procedure by which lymph nodes can be removed for microscopic examination.

**Mediastinum**: Area between the lungs.

**Metastasis**: The spread of cancer from the initial cancer site to other parts of the body.

**Minimally invasive surgery**: Surgery which uses smaller incisions than a regular operation and thus is less painful for the patient post-operatively. In order to be able to operate through such a small incision, the surgeon must use advanced, fibro electronic instruments.

**Mortality**: The number of people who die of a disease.

**Multidisciplinary clinic**: A multidisciplinary clinic is one in which doctors of different specialities (e.g., medical oncology, radiation oncology, and surgeons) all see the patient within the same clinic.

**Mutation**: Damage in the DNA. Depending on the mutation and where it is located, it may result in cancer. Cancer-causing mutations are often due to carcinogens (cancer causing substances)such as substances found in the diet or cigarette smoke. Some mutations may be inherited (usually not in lung cancer). There are many different types of mutations (deletions, insertions, amplifications, translocations, gene rearrangements, etc.).

**Myelosuppression**: A decrease in the production of blood cells.

# N

**N2 nodes**: Mediastinal nodes (e.g., nodes between the lungs and the heart).

**Nicotine replacement therapy**: Smoking cessation method that uses nicotine substitutes in various forms, including a patch, gum, inhaler, or nasal spray.

**Non-small cell lung cancer (NSCLC)**: A type of lung cancer that includes adenocarcinoma, squamous cell carcinoma, and large cell carcinoma.

**Nucleus**: The area of a cell where the DNA resides.

**P**

**Palliative treatment**: Treatment given not with the intent to cure but with the intent to prolong survival and reduce symptoms from the tumor.

**Pancoast tumor (superior sulcus tumor)**: A tumor occurring near the top of the lungs that may cause shoulder pain or weakness or a group of symptoms including a droopy eyelid, dry eyes, and lack of sweating on the face.

**Parietal pleura**: A membrane lining the chest wall.

**Passive smoking**: Inhaling cigarette smoke of others.

**Patient-controlled analgesia (PCA)**: A method by which a patient can regulate the amount of pain medication he or she receives.

**PD1**: A substance found on T-cells which can bind to PD-L1. Once bound, the T-cell does not recognize the foreign intruder. It becomes inactivated, and in turn does not activate the rest of the immune system.

**PD-L1**: A substance made by some normal cells to turn off the immune system. It works by binding to PD-1 on T cells. Some cancers cells also make PD-L1.

**Pericardial effusion**: Accumulation of fluid inside the sac (pericardium) that surrounds the heart.

**Pericardium**: A double-layered serous membrane that surrounds the heart.

**Phlebotomist**: A technician trained to draw blood.

**Placebo**: An inactive substance (e.g., sugar pill). Placebos alone are rarely used in cancer trials.

**Pleural catheter**: Provides symptomatic relief of dyspnea related to recurrent pleural effusions.

**Pleural effusion**: Accumulation of fluid between the outside of the lung and the inside of the chest wall.

**Pleural space**: The area between the outside of the lung and the inside of the chest wall.

**Pleurodesis**: A procedure to prevent recurrence of pleural effusion by draining the fluid and inserting medication into the pleural space.

**Pneumonectomy**: Surgical removal of the entire lung.

**Pneumonia**: An infection of the lung.

**Pneumonitis**: Irritation of the lungs.

**Poorly differentiated**: Cancer cells that look wildly abnormal and nothing like the organ they started in.

**Pulmonary function tests (PFTs):** A group of breathing tests used to determine lung health.

**Pulmonologist:** A physician who specializes in the diagnosis and treatment of lung diseases.

## R

**Radiation therapy:** Treatment that uses high-dose X-rays or other high-energy rays to kill cancer cells.

**Radioprotectant:** A medication that reduces certain side effects of radiation.

**Radiotherapy:** The treatment of disease with ionizing radiation. Also called **radiation therapy**.

**Rads:** A deprecated unit of absorbed radiation dose, defined as 1 rad = 0.01 Gy – 0.01 J/kg.

**Randomized controlled trial (RCT):** A research study in which the participants are assigned by chance (using a computer) to separate groups that compare different treatments; a method used to prevent bias in research.

**Receptor:** A protein molecule, embedded in either the plasma membrane or cytoplasm of a cell, to which a signaling molecule (or ligand) may attach.

**Regimen:** Specific chemotherapy treatment plan involving the drugs, doses, and frequency of administration.

**Resectable:** Able to be surgically removed (resected).

**Resection:** Surgical removal.

**Respiratory depression:** Slowing of breathing.

**Robotic surgery:** A type of minimally invasive surgery, in which the surgeon manipulates the instruments from a console that does not have to be next to the patient's bed.

## S

**Sequencing:** A way of looking at the DNA of the genes to find out if they are normal or not.

**Small cell carcinoma:** A type of lung cancer that differs in appearance and behavior from non-small cell lung cancers (adenocarcinoma, squamous cell carcinoma, large cell carcinoma).

**Small cell lung cancer (SCLC):** Refers to small cell carcinoma, as opposed to non-small cell lung cancers (adenocarcinoma, squamous cell carcinoma, large cell carcinoma).

**Sputum:** Mucus and other secretions produced by the lungs.

**Squamous cell carcinoma**: A type of non-small cell lung cancer.

**Staging**: Determining the size of a cancer and how far it has spread.

**Stent**: A hollow tube that can be inserted via bronchoscopy into the airway to prevent it from being blocked or crushed by the tumor.

**Superior sulcus tumor**: See pancoast tumor.

**Superior vena cava syndrome (SVCS)**: A collection of symptoms that could include swelling in the neck, shoulders, and arms caused by a lung tumor pressing on the SVC, one of the large vessels leading into the heart.

**Surgery**: Removal of tissue by means of an operation (surgical procedure).

**Systemic**: Affecting the entire body.

**T**

**T-lymphocytes (T cells)**: A type of white blood cell which is important in recognizing an abnormal substance, such as viruses, bacteria, or cancer cells, and then activating the rest of the immune system.

**Targeted therapy**: Therapy directed at aspects of the cell that are specific for cancer.

**Thoracentesis**: A procedure that uses a needle to remove fluid from the space between the lung and the chest wall.

**Thoracotomy**: A common type of lung surgery that requires a large incision to provide access to the lungs.

**Trachea**: Breathing tube (airway) leading from the larynx to the lungs.

**Transthoracic (percutaneous) biopsy**: A biopsy in which a needle is inserted from the outside into the tumor.

**Tumor**: A mass of tissue formed by a new growth of cells.

**Tyrosine kinase inhibitors (TKIs)**: Small molecules which block the activated part of the receptor on the inside of the cancer cell and prevent it from starting a chemical reaction which causes the cell to grow and divide.

**V**

**VEGF (vascular endothelial growth factor)**: A family of growth factors, most often made by tumors, that causes blood vessel cells (vascular cells) to grow into the tumor.

**Video-assisted thoracoscopic surgery (VATS)**: A type of minimally invasive chest surgery.

**Visceral pleura**: A membrane surrounding the lung.

## W

**Wedge resection**: Surgical removal of the tumor and a small amount of lung tissue surrounding the tumor.

**Well-differentiated**: Cancer cells which look relatively similar to the organ in which they started.

**White blood cells**: A type of blood cell that fights infection.

## X

**X-ray**: High-energy radiation used to image the body.

INDEX